EFFECTIVE PSYCHOTHERAPISTS

Also Available

Effective Psychotherapists

CLINICAL SKILLS
THAT IMPROVE CLIENT OUTCOMES

William R. Miller
Theresa B. Moyers

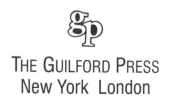

THE GUILFORD PRESS
New York London

Copyright © 2021 The Guilford Press
A Division of Guilford Publications, Inc.
370 Seventh Avenue, Suite 1200, New York, NY 10001
www.guilford.com

Printed in the United States of America

This book is printed on acid-free paper.

Last digit is print number: 9   8   7   6   5   4   3

The authors have checked with sources believed to be reliable in their
efforts to provide information that is complete and generally in accord
with the standards of practice that are accepted at the time of publication.
However, in view of the possibility of human error or changes in behavioral,
mental health, or medical sciences, neither the authors, nor the editor and
publisher, nor any other party who has been involved in the preparation
or publication of this work warrants that the information contained herein
is in every respect accurate or complete, and they are not responsible
for any errors or omissions or the results obtained from the use of such
information. Readers are encouraged to confirm the information contained
in this book with other sources.

Library of Congress Cataloging-in-Publication Data
is available from the publisher.

ISBN 978-1-4625-4689-3 (paperback) 978-1-4625-4535-3 (hardcover)

For my wife, Kathy Jackson,
who continues to teach me about loving relationships
—WRM

For my mother, Ruth Aiken Ellett,
who was my first and most powerful teacher
in the value of genuineness
—TBM

About the Authors

William R. Miller, PhD, is Emeritus Distinguished Professor of Psychology and Psychiatry at the University of New Mexico. Fundamentally interested in the psychology of change, he is a cofounder of motivational interviewing (MI) and has focused particularly on developing and testing more effective treatments for people with alcohol and drug problems. Dr. Miller has published over 400 scientific articles and chapters and 60 books, including the groundbreaking work for professionals *Motivational Interviewing, Third Edition,* and the self-help resource *Controlling Your Drinking, Second Edition.* He is a recipient of the international Jellinek Memorial Award, two career achievement awards from the American Psychological Association, and an Innovators in Combating Substance Abuse Award from the Robert Wood Johnson Foundation, among many other honors. The Institute for Scientific Information has listed him as one of the world's most highly cited researchers.

Theresa B. Moyers, PhD, is Associate Professor of Psychology at the University of New Mexico, where she conducts research on treatments for addictive behaviors, with a focus on MI. Her primary interests are identifying the active ingredients of MI as well as optimal methods for disseminating it in addictions settings. Dr. Moyers has published more than 35 peer-reviewed articles and has presented on MI and addictions treatment in 16 countries. She is a member of the Motivational Interviewing Network of Trainers. In addition to her academic pursuits, she trains and competes with her border collie in the sport of dog agility. Her website is *www.theresamoyers.com*.

Preface

Perhaps the best way to start is with the story of how this book emerged. The seeds for it were planted long ago through a series of happenstance events, several of which occurred during my predoctoral psychology training at the University of Oregon. The clinical program at Oregon was strongly behavioral, and even "cognitive-behavioral" was a new and controversial concept in the early 1970s. Students at Oregon normally didn't begin seeing clients until the third year of training, after we had done the heavy lifting of coursework and a master's thesis. During the second year, there was a required two-semester seminar to prepare us for talking to clients, and apparently none of the behaviorists wanted to teach it, so they found a faculty member from the Counseling Psychology Department to prepare us for clinical work. Mentored by Leona Tyler and thus an academic grandchild of Carl Rogers, Sue Gilmore introduced us to a person-centered way of listening to and being with clients before we ever set foot in the practice of behavior therapy.

Clinical practica began in our third year, and I joined one that focused on family therapy, supervised by Steve Johnson. Steve's own mentor, Gerald Patterson, was a progenitor of behavioral family therapy who had been on the clinical faculty but had moved across town to the Oregon Research Institute (ORI). I was working with families in the university psychology clinic, trying to follow the guidelines in

Patterson's writings, teaching parents about positive reinforcement and behavior tracking, but without much success. Then we took a field trip over to ORI to watch (via a one-way mirror) Patterson working with a family. He was indeed using the techniques he had described, but he was doing much more than what was mentioned in his writing. He was a warm, empathic, patient, funny, engaging human being. "So *that's* how you do it," I thought. Back in the clinic, I began following his example and integrating what we had learned about a client-centered approach. I found parents more engaged in the treatment process, more willing to try the homework assignments that I suggested, and more successful with the behavior changes for which they hoped (Miller & Danaher, 1976). It was not until decades later that I encountered this quote: "It should be reemphasized that, in spite of the cold and mechanistic language used to describe [behavior therapy] techniques, the actual practice often involves a warm, authentic, and deeply understanding therapist" (Truax & Carkhuff, 1967, p. 360).

Just before my third year of graduate training, I had a summer internship on the alcoholism ward at the Veterans Administration hospital in Milwaukee, Wisconsin. Fortunately, I knew nothing about alcoholism, so being a newcomer, I spent most of the summer listening with the same Rogerian skills that I had learned. The clients taught me about alcoholism, and both they and I enjoyed the conversations. I also began learning some behavior therapies that summer and decided to focus my dissertation on treating people with alcohol problems (Miller, 1978). The outcomes were good, with an unexpected twist. At the end of treatment, clients (randomly chosen) either received or did not receive a self-help booklet describing the same methods our counselors were using. During subsequent follow-up, clients who had been given the book showed a significant further decrease in their drinking, whereas the others did not. This unexpected finding suggested a second study was in order, one in which problem drinkers were randomly assigned to receive the 10-session outpatient behavior therapy we had developed, or were instead seen for just one session, given the self-help book, and encouraged to use it. To our surprise, both groups showed the same large reduction in alcohol use, with no difference between groups (Miller, Gribskov, & Mortell, 1981). With or without ongoing counselor support, both groups changed their long-standing drinking patterns.

I joined the clinical psychology faculty at the University of New Mexico in 1976 and continued this line of research, training counselors in both client-centered and behavior therapies. Three times we replicated in randomized trials the finding that clients, on average, fared just as well when working on their own with our self-help guidebook (Miller & Muñoz, 1976) as when treated by a counselor using the same methods. In one of these studies (Miller, Taylor, & West, 1980), three supervisors observed therapy sessions (again via one-way mirrors; this was before we could afford video equipment) both for adherence to behavior therapy techniques and for the quality of empathic listening skills (Truax & Carkhuff, 1967). We independently ranked the therapists on their skill in accurate empathy, with excellent interrater agreement. When the follow-up data came in, we examined differences in clients' outcomes across therapists. Again to our surprise, we found that we could strongly predict clients' subsequent drinking from how well their behavior therapist had *listened* to them! At 6-month follow-up, the most empathic counselor had a 100% success rate, and the least empathic of the nine therapists had a 25% success rate. *On average,* counselors' success rate was 61%, as compared with 60% for those working on their own with self-help materials. This might lead one to conclude that therapists are no different from self-help, but, in fact, five therapists had success rates of 75% or higher, whereas for three counselors it appeared that clients would have been better off going home with a good book. Even 2 years after treatment had ended, counselor empathy still significantly predicted clients' drinking outcomes (Miller & Baca, 1983). Therapeutic relationship mattered, whereas there were no outcome differences among the specific behavioral techniques that we were comparing. In a later study (Miller, Benefield, & Tonigan, 1993), we were able to predict clients' alcohol use 12 months after treatment from the *opposite* of empathic listening: The more therapists confronted, the more their clients drank.

The message that I was clearly receiving from our data is that it matters greatly *how* you counsel. The person-centered approach of Carl Rogers formed a foundation for the method of motivational interviewing that I first described in 1983 through discussions and experiential practice with a group of Norwegian psychologists, and have been refining ever since. For three decades in our predoctoral clinical program, I taught the first-semester course on how to talk with clients, focusing initially on Rogers's person-centered counseling skills and later more broadly on motivational interviewing.

Skip ahead a few years: In retirement, I decided to revisit the classic volume written by two of Rogers's students (Truax & Carkhuff, 1967). A surprise for me was that they were not really promoting yet another competing method of psychotherapy. Rogers's explanatory theory was virtually unmentioned. They were interested not in creating a new school of therapy, but rather in developing better *therapists,* explicitly exploring how the relational insights of Rogers might be integrated with behavioral therapies. This had eluded me before. I'd spent a good bit of my career arguing for the preferential use of evidence-based treatment methods for alcohol use disorders. I do still believe, as Rogers did, that we must pay attention to what scientific research tells us about what works and what doesn't. It was Rogers, in fact, who played a key role in bringing clinical psychology into the American Psychological Association and the mainstream of scientific psychology (Kirschenbaum, 2009; Miller & Moyers, 2017). "Believe your data" is one of the few things about which Carl Rogers and B. F. Skinner agreed. What I had missed is the emphasis on the qualities of counselors and therapists themselves that improve clients' outcomes regardless of the treatment method being used.

Following our own data is what led to this book, and I am delighted that Terri Moyers agreed to accompany me on the journey. Her research has faithfully followed in the footsteps of Rogers and his students, patiently using painstaking methodologies to understand important processes in the therapeutic relationship and how they impact treatment outcome. We understand that these interpersonal processes apply far beyond counseling and psychotherapy, affecting the quality and outcomes of teaching, health care, coaching, and many other helping relationships. We happen to have studied them in the context of psychological treatment, which is our primary focus in this volume.

Our own clinical research has focused more specifically on the treatment of addictive behaviors, a life-and-death field that has fascinated and never bored me since my 1973 initiation in Milwaukee. A definite scientific advantage of working in addiction treatment is that there is a clear behavioral outcome measure. To be sure, there are other important dimensions of recovery, but if you haven't had an impact on your client's substance use or other addictive behavior, you probably haven't helped much. When treating schizophrenia, the Rogers group had to rely on global outcome measures such as MMPI scales and clinician ratings of functioning to evaluate their efforts. A more specific outcome measure (such as substance use) allows for closer study of process–outcome relationships. The therapist attributes that are the focus of this book did not begin with and are by no means limited to treating addiction. It's just that addiction is such a clear lens through which to study and understand the psychology of change (DiClemente, 2003).

In essence, what we are attempting in this book is an update, over half a century later, of the classic Truax and Carkhuff volume *Toward Effective Counseling and Psychotherapy*. Much has changed in helping professions during the ensuing decades. Despite the solid research and warnings in their two volumes (Truax & Carkhuff, 1967, 1976), clinical psychology, in particular, seems fixated on specific treatment techniques, whereas Truax and Carkhuff asserted, "The central question to be asked in counseling and psychotherapy is 'What are the essential characteristics or behaviors of the therapist or counselor that lead to constructive behavioral change in the client?'" (1967, p. 24).

In clinical trials, therapist effects are often regarded as nuisance noise that compromises therapeutic effect size, rather than as an important component in effective treatment. We believe Rogers and his students were on the right track in their research. Therapist relational factors have too often been overlooked in mainstream clinical research and training. We do not discount the potential importance of specific treatment procedures with particular disorders. At the same time, evidence-based treatments cannot be separated from the therapists who deliver them. For those looking for important clinical research topics, the chapters ahead may suggest a wealth of options.

About Language

Because the relational dimensions that we discuss apply to so many helping professions, it was a challenge to decide what terms to use to describe service providers. In the end, we stayed mostly with generic terms like "counselor," "clinician," and "therapist," although these apply less well to helpers such as teachers and coaches. Similarly, one must decide how to describe the recipients of helping services. Again, we could not improve on the generic term "client" (or in explicitly medical contexts, "patient") and sometimes just "people." Thus, we stayed close to the terminology used by Rogers, Truax, and Carkhuff.

We anticipate that many readers of this book will come from behavioral health professions, and therein lies another language issue. Whereas "behavioral" once connoted therapies derived from learning theory with philosophic overtones of behaviorism, it now applies more broadly as "behavioral science." Counseling and psychotherapy are described generically as "behavioral" (as distinct, e.g., from pharmacological). More generally, efforts to support psychological well-being are termed "behavioral health," replacing the earlier term "mental health." That is our generic intention when using the term "behavioral" in this volume, whereas we use "behavior therapy" when we mean to refer specifically to interventions focusing more on behavior and drawing on learning theory.

With that said, we hope our work will also be useful in helping relationships well beyond counseling and psychotherapy. Interpersonal dynamics affect the course and outcomes of human interactions. We have been fortunate to study and use them within the discipline of psychology, but we find that what we have learned does apply in life and relationships more broadly, and is vital in healing and helping professions.

WILLIAM R. MILLER
Albuquerque, New Mexico

Contents

PART III. LEARNING, TRAINING, AND CLINICAL SCIENCE

PART I

HELPING RELATIONSHIPS

What is important in treatment? Is it the specific techniques being used, or is it the quality of therapeutic relationship? There is no reason to believe that it must be one or the other. In surgery, for example, outcomes vary by the particular procedures being used and also by the skillfulness of the surgeon using them.

In this volume, we focus on what is known about the skills of therapists themselves that influence client outcomes. Chapter 1 invites you to consider how therapists' skills and attitudes affect outcomes for better or worse across a broad range of treatment methods and theoretical orientations. How much do these counselor qualities affect clients' outcomes? In Chapter 2, we summarize and discuss the large clinical research literature on this very question.

An Invitation

Counseling and psychotherapy are inseparable from the people who provide them. Within almost any psychological treatment, clients' outcomes vary widely depending on the person who treats them. What is it that renders some therapists so much more effective than others, even when they are delivering the same highly structured treatment? That is the question at the heart of this book.

We have been committed to improving clients' outcomes, as well as helping behavioral health providers continue to enjoy and grow professionally in their work. For therapists, that does not happen automatically in the context of ongoing practice. A distressing and well-replicated finding in psychotherapy research is that therapists (unlike surgeons) usually do not get better with practice (Budge et al., 2013; Erekson, Janis, Bailey, Cattani, & Pedersen, 2017; Norton & Little, 2014; M. L. Smith, Glass, & Miller, 1980; Tracey, Wampold, Lichtenberg, & Goodyear, 2014). Why is that? In Chapter 12, we will explore how this may be a function of the normal conditions of clinical practice (Dawes, 1994).

> *Counseling and psychotherapy are inseparable from the people who provide them.*

The good news is that there is something you can do to continue developing therapeutic expertise after initial training.

Therapeutic Skills

If there is a consensus among major theories of psychotherapy, it is the importance of a good "working alliance," a solid therapeutic relationship (Flückiger et al., in press). One assertion is that more effective therapists (those whose clients tend to get better) share certain interpersonal characteristics regardless of their particular theoretical orientation or treatment approach (T. Anderson, Ogles, Patterson, Lambert, & Vermeersch, 2009; Okiishi, Lambert, Nielsen, & Ogles, 2003). This is not a new idea. In 1967, Charles Truax and Robert Carkhuff published their groundbreaking book *Toward Effective Counseling and Psychotherapy.* They were not seeking to promote a particular school of psychotherapy. Rather, they sought to understand what it is that more effective counselors actually *do* so that training could focus on developing better *therapists.* They pulled together an already large body of research, pioneering the measurement and training of active ingredients of psychotherapy such as empathy, warmth, and acceptance that have sometimes been termed "common" or "nonspecific" factors.

It can be misleading to call these "common" factors, which suggests that they are present in all delivered therapies. In fact, practitioners vary widely in relational characteristics such as accurate empathy and warmth. It has long been known that therapeutic factors like acceptance, warmth, and empathy are not actually "common" in the sense of widespread or universal. Hans Strupp (1960) found that fewer than 5 percent of 2,474 responses from 126 psychiatrists in five cities reflected even mild interpersonal warmth. Six decades later, a study of social work practice similarly found that a high level of empathy was uncommon (Lynch, Newlands, & Forrester, 2019). Furthermore, to refer to these as "nonspecific" factors is to confess that we have not done our homework, for as Truax and Carkhuff amply demonstrated half a century ago, such factors can be specified, reliably measured, studied, and taught. They also documented that therapist factors like accurate empathy do matter; they predict client outcomes. In psychology, the roots of modern clinical science lie in this early work of Carl Rogers and his students on therapeutic mechanisms and outcomes (Miller & Moyers, 2017). We prefer the convention of referring to these as *therapeutic* skills, factors, or conditions (Frank, 1971; Kivlighan & Holmes, 2004).

There is extensive evidence to indicate that these therapeutic factors do facilitate better client outcomes across a broad range of treatment methods and contexts. They are *ways* of doing what else you do in practice. These are not personality traits, but interpersonal skills that can be improved over time.

Furthermore, these factors are directly related to what therapists often find to be most rewarding about their work (Larson, 2020). Behavioral health professions tend to attract those who enjoy talking with and getting to know a wide range of people. What engages therapists is not usually the mastery of particular techniques, but the privilege of relating to people at a level of depth and intimacy well beyond ordinary social discourse.

Therapeutic conditions are interpersonal skills that can be improved over time.

Clinical training, however, too often focuses on learning specific knowledge and technique, with relatively little attention to the therapeutic skills that have at least as much impact on client outcomes as the specific treatment methods being used.

Mind and Heart: Therapeutic Attitudes

Throughout this book, we will be describing how interpersonal therapeutic skills involve both an internal *experiential* component and an external *expressive* component. Rogers (1980a) referred to the experiential elements as therapist "attitudes," and Truax and Carkhuff (1967, 1976) advanced the behavioral measurement and practice of the expressive components. Practice influences attitude, and vice versa.

There are many descriptions of important therapeutic attitudes underlying counseling and psychotherapy (Fromm, 1956; Miller, 2017; Miller & Rollnick, 2013; Rogers, 1980d; Yalom, 2002). Perhaps most fundamental in helping relationships is a commitment to *compassion*. This is not just "feeling for" (sympathy), but a desire and intention to alleviate suffering and facilitate others' wellness and growth (Armstrong, 2010; Fromm, 1956; The Dalai Lama & Vreeland, 2001). A helping relationship is not for the helper's benefit; the prime directive is the client's well-being. In this way, helping relationships differ from friendship and intimate relationships, where ideally both partners have a mutual commitment to promoting each other's health and wellness. Compassionate beneficence underlies all of the therapeutic skills to be discussed in Part II of this book, and is codified in the professional ethical standards of helping professions such as medicine, social work, and psychology.

A second therapeutic attitude underlying therapeutic skills is a sense of counseling and psychotherapy as a *partnership*. Some kinds of interventions are delivered not by a collaborator but by an expert to a passive patient. For example, a surgeon operates on an anesthetized person to excise a tumor. A dentist removes and replaces decayed tooth tissue. At an accident scene, a paramedic performs cardiopulmonary resuscitation and stops the bleeding. A lifeguard rescues a floundering swimmer. A physician prescribes the correct antibiotic for an infection. At most, what is required of the recipient of such services is "patient" cooperation.

Most helping relationships are not like this. The work of teachers, coaches, health educators, mentors, counselors, and therapists usually focuses on behavior, broadly speaking: on what people do, how they think and relate to others. Addictions, chronic illnesses, and criminal behavior are very much about lifestyle. If the helping goal is to change people's behavior or lifestyle, you simply cannot *make* them change in the way that a dentist extracts a faulty tooth, or a surgeon excises a malignant tumor. Human beings make their own choices about what they will do and how they will live, and efforts to persuade or coerce change can have an unintended opposite effect (Brehm & Brehm, 1981; de Almeida Neto, 2017; Karno & Longabaugh, 2005). Even the success of a heroic acute intervention often depends ultimately on the person's subsequent behavior. Surgeons lament that so many patients do not follow through with needed action (like wound care and physical rehabilitation). No matter how impressive the technical skills of a professional, the active participation of the human recipient of care is almost always required for the best outcomes when behavior is involved.

In order to help people change their behavior or lifestyle, you need *their* expertise and partnership. No one knows more about your clients than they do. They have a lifetime of experience to draw on. You do bring professional expertise that may be helpful, but you cannot be an expert on someone else's life. A helping relationship is not a matter of an expert doing something *to* or using techniques *on* clients. It is about working *with, alongside,* and *for* clients. It is not like wrestling; it's more like dancing together (Miller & Rollnick, 2013).

In Part II, we will invite you to consider eight therapeutic skills that can improve your clients' outcomes. It is probably easiest to focus on developing one of these therapeutic skills at a time. Benjamin Franklin (2012/1785) described a set of 13 personal virtues, including some behavioral descriptions and a method for self-monitoring (cf. Brooks, 2015). Rather than seeking to strengthen them all together, he decided to focus intentionally on each of them for one week at a time. This created a cycle of 13 weeks that he could repeat four times a year. He also recommended choosing an order of practice so that successive virtues would build on each other. To some extent, we arranged the chapters of Part II in that way, with accurate empathy (Chapter 3) forming a foundation on which other skills such as acceptance and affirmation can be built.

Finally, in Part III, we will discuss the learning (Chapter 12) and teaching of therapeutic skills (Chapter 13), and reflect on some implications for a broader clinical science (Chapter 14). Before proceeding, however, we devote Chapter 2 to a question underlying all of this: How much do therapists really matter in treatment? The answer may surprise you.

KEY POINTS

- Counseling and psychotherapy are inseparable from the people who provide them.
- Psychotherapists do not automatically get better with practice.
- More effective therapists (regardless of their treatment approach) share certain interpersonal characteristics that can be specified, measured, learned, and practiced.
- Therapeutic skills have both an internal *experiential* component and an external *expressive* component.
- Compassion and partnership are broad therapeutic attitudes underlying the therapeutic skills.
- To help people change their behavior or lifestyle, you need *their* expertise and active engagement.

CHAPTER 2

Therapist Effects

Behavioral treatment outcome research has often been conducted as though therapists don't matter and are interchangeable. Specific manual-guided therapies are often presumed to be the same no matter who provides them. Is it so?

Research on Therapist Effects

Therapist effects have been a subject of psychological research since the 1940s, and the results have been reassuringly consistent over time. Newer and better-designed studies are telling the same story as their older counterparts: There are important differences among therapists in their clients' outcomes, for better or worse, and these differences have to do with interpersonal therapeutic skills.

One study of the impact of therapist skills across time in a clinical setting found that postgraduate trainees with better interpersonal skills at baseline also had better client outcomes *across 5 years* (Schottke, Fluckiger, Goldberg, Eversmann, & Lange, 2017). The difference remained after controlling for any impact of theoretical orientation, client and therapist characteristics, and amount of supervision. Other studies have similarly found that a counselor's therapeutic skills predict client outcomes, whereas other therapist characteristics (such as years of experience and theoretical orientation) do not (e.g., T. Anderson, McClintock, Himawan, Song, & Patterson, 2016; T. Anderson et al., 2009; Pfeiffer et al., 2020). Thomas Haug and colleagues (2016) found that both interpersonal skills and technical skills made independent contributions to outcomes for clients with social anxiety. We similarly found that both therapist empathy and the specific content of behavior therapy were associated with better outcomes for clients with alcohol use disorders (Moyers, Houck, Rice, Longabaugh, & Miller, 2016).

There are important differences among therapists in their clients' outcomes.

A study that stretched the limits of what it means to be a therapist (T. Anderson, Crowley, Himawan, Holmberg, & Uhlin, 2016) evaluated the interpersonal skills of 23 graduate student interventionists, 11 of whom were in a clinical psychology program, and 12 others with no prior clinical training, coming from other disciplines like chemistry, biology, and history. All of the interventionists were evaluated for therapeutic interpersonal skills (including empathy, sociability, and social skills) and then randomly assigned to clients (who were students experiencing distress but not necessarily seeking therapy). They found that "therapists" higher in baseline interpersonal skills had better client improvement across all outcome measures, regardless of their academic discipline. In other words, interpersonal skills were a better predictor of outcome than whether the therapists were studying psychology or another field.

Therapists versus Other Factors

How much of a difference do therapists make in the big picture? One approach is to ask how important therapists are compared to all of the other elements that matter in a course of treatment. (This is called a "random effects model.") Using a cooking analogy: How much does the quality of meals depend on the chef, compared to the ingredients being used, the recipes, conditions in the kitchen, the type of restaurant, the customers, and the season of the year? In treatment outcome research, such other factors include attributes of the clients being treated (e.g., age, gender, problem severity, personality), of the treatment itself (e.g., length, structure, manual-guided, supervision, and quality assurance), of the setting (e.g., residential or outpatient, correctional, faith-based, fee structure), and of the providers (e.g., education, experience, personality, interpersonal skills).

Studies of this kind typically find little or no outcome difference based on the specific treatments being compared, but a significant difference attributable to the therapists who provided the treatments. This is true for two of the most common behavioral diagnoses: depression (Kim, Wampold, & Bolt, 2006; Zuroff, Kelly, Leybman, Blatt, & Wampold, 2010) and substance use disorders (Imel, Wampold, Miller, & Fleming, 2008; Miller, Forcehimes, & Zweben, 2019; Project MATCH Research Group, 1997, 1998). Similarly, one of the largest naturalistic therapy studies ever done examined the outcomes for 6,146 clients who had been assigned to 581 therapists for a variety of problems in a managed care setting (Wampold & Brown, 2005). Significant differences in outcome were attributable to therapists, and this variability was not explained by the therapists' age, gender, professional experience, or degree. In this same study, there was no effect at all for the specific kind of treatment that clients received.

It is also possible for both therapists and specific interventions to have independent effects on client outcomes. A study with 38 therapists and 700 clients examined the contributions of therapists and their skills as well as specific cognitive-behavioral therapy modules to outcomes in the treatment of alcohol use disorders (Moyers, Houck, et al., 2016). Three specific components of the behavioral intervention were associated with improved client outcomes: mood management, coping with craving and urges, and social and recreational counseling. Therapists also contributed substantially to outcomes, with higher expression of therapist empathy (Chapter 3) predicting greater reduction in alcohol use. "Relatively small increases in the therapist's usual level of empathy were associated with larger decreases in end-of-treatment drinking" (Moyers et al., 2016, p. 226). This finding is noteworthy in that all therapists had been prescreened to have at least moderate competence with empathic skills, and their treatment sessions (including expression of empathy) were closely monitored throughout the trial. There was no significant interaction between therapists and treatments. In other words, both therapists and treatment procedures mattered independently from each other.

It is possible for both therapists and specific interventions to have independent effects on client outcomes.

Differences between Therapists

What about comparing therapists to each other when all clients in a study are receiving the same kinds of treatment or, as in a natural setting, are getting treatment as usual? (This is called a "fixed effects model.") Is a client better off being treated by one therapist rather than another, or are all therapists about the same? When two chefs are working with the same ingredients, how different will their meals be?

The answer here is startlingly clear. There are often large differences among therapists who are offering the same or similar treatments, and those differences predict client outcomes and are consistent over time (Kraus et al., 2016; Owen et al, 2019). When such studies are conducted in naturalistic settings like a managed care organization (rather than in psychotherapy research laboratories), the effects are larger still, perhaps because there is greater variability in the kinds of therapists employed in real-world settings. Differences in therapist effectiveness can be detected as early as the first session, predicting clients' treatment outcomes (Erekson, Clayson, Park, & Tass, 2020).

For example, in a study at a large university counseling center, outcomes for 1,841 clients were studied over a 30-month period (Okiishi et al., 2003). Clients were assigned to therapists based on who had an open slot in their calendar (i.e., as randomly as is likely feasible in a real-world setting). There were no significant differences among therapists in the initial severity level of their clients. Clients completed questionnaires weekly to track their improvement, and 91 therapists were then rank-ordered according to their clients' outcomes. The three top-ranked therapists saw clients for an average of 2.4 sessions, with an improvement rate 8 times greater than average in this counseling center. The three lowest-ranked therapists saw clients for three times as long (7.9 sessions on average), with symptoms worsening on average. Large differences among therapists have been common in other studies (Kim et al., 2006; Luborsky, McLellan, Diguer, Woody, & Seligman, 1997; Moyers, Houck, et al., 2016) and are abundant in addiction treatment research (Luborsky, McLellan, Woody, O'Brien, & Auerbach, 1985; Miller, Taylor, & West, 1980; Valle, 1981).

A sobering finding of studies comparing therapists to each other is that some therapists, rather than simply being ineffective, may actually be harming their clients. It has often been assumed that psychotherapy is a benign process in which the worst outcome would be that clients do not benefit. In fact, therapists (and therapies) can cause harm. In one clinical trial, a single clinician accounted for most of the overall therapist effect; at follow-up, nearly all of this therapist's clients were drinking daily (Project MATCH Research Group, 1998). In a series of studies with schizophrenic clients (Rogers, Gendlin, Kiesler, & Truax, 1967), therapists who were low in empathy and unconditional positive regard were more likely to have clients who were deteriorating rather than improving—again a common finding (Moyers & Miller, 2013). Charles Truax and Robert Carkhuff (1967) urged that "the various related professions should take an active hand in weeding out or retraining therapists, educators, counselors, etc., who are unable to provide high levels of effective ingredients, and who therefore are likely to provide human encounters that change people *for the worse*" (p. 142, italics in the original). More than half a century later, harm from psychotherapy remains relatively unexplored in clinical research (Dimidjian & Hollon, 2010), and those who train, supervise, and study behavioral health providers have rarely grappled effectively with toxic therapists (Castonguay, Boswell, Constantino, Goldfried, & Hill, 2010). Counselors who are harming their clients are unlikely to realize it themselves, nor will the systems within which they work detect the harm unless providers' outcomes are monitored. Removing a few therapists with the poorest outcomes could substantially improve an agency's or system's overall results while diminishing the likelihood of harm to clients (Imel, Sheng, Baldwin, & Atkins, 2015).

Some therapists, rather than simply being ineffective, may actually be harming their clients.

Differences within Therapists

Considering the strength of evidence supporting therapist effects, it would be easy to conclude that individual providers consistently have a beneficial (or harmful) effect no matter which clients they are seeing. This is not so. Therapists do differ in overall effectiveness (i.e., can be rank-ordered in their helpfulness when compared with each other) *and also* vary in their skills and effectiveness depending on the clients they are treating. Even the best therapists are not effective with every client, and even the worst may be helpful with a few. Some of what explains therapists' success lies in their interaction with different clients.

For example, the overall level of empathy measured in treatment sessions often differs between therapists (see Chapter 3), and clients are more likely, on average, to improve when working with therapists who have stronger empathic skills. However, there is also significant variability in the quality of empathy among a therapist's treatment sessions for different clients, and this variability also predicts outcome. It is not only the *average* level of empathy a therapist shows that is important, but also how much empathy is evident in any particular session. In fact, this within-caseload variability usually accounts for more variance in outcomes than do the differences between therapists. This suggests an important "give and take" between therapist and client in how their interaction accounts for better (or worse) results. Therapists (and their supervisors) ought to be interested in not only how good their therapeutic skills are on average, but also how and why they vary in the expression of these skills with different clients. Therapists' overall skills are

> *Even the best therapists are not effective with every client, and even the worst may be helpful with a few.*

important, and so is their ability to adapt how they use those skills with clients who vary in many ways.

Client–Therapist Match

This raises a question to keep in mind as we consider specific therapeutic skills in the chapters of Part II. How can conscientious therapists identify and respond to client characteristics that affect their own talents and skills? Some of the relevant client attributes may be similar across most therapists. A familiar adage is that therapists tend to prefer clients who are young, attractive, verbal, intelligent, and successful (YAVIS) more than those who are older, plain, quiet, average, and struggling (Kugelmass, 2016; Schofield, 1964; Teasdale & Hill, 2006). There will be other biases that therapists harbor in working with various clients, and demographic client variables such as age, ethnicity, and gender do not tell the whole story. Experienced therapists know it is easier to form a collaboration with some clients than with others, for reasons that are not always clear.

Research indicates that the fit between client characteristics and therapist skills can matter. For example, clients with more externalizing symptoms (such as substance use) appear to respond better when treatments are focused on their symptoms, whereas those with internalizing symptoms (such as anxiety and depression) are more amenable to a search for insight (Beutler, Kimpara, Edwards, & Miller, 2018). Similarly, more directive therapists (and therapies) may work better with clients who are lower in anger and reactance (Karno & Longabaugh, 2005; Waldron, Miller, & Tonigan, 2001). It is possible, however, for therapists to vary in their expression of therapeutic skills across clients and even within the same client's sessions over time, responding to a host of variables of which they may be only partially aware.

Therapies and Therapists

What matters in counseling and psychotherapy? Is it the specific treatment techniques used, or the therapists who are providing them (Blow, Sprenkle, & Davis, 2007)? Returning to our culinary analogy: What makes a good meal? Is it the chef, or the raw ingredients? The illusion lies in the word "or" —that it must be one or the other. Both matter. Specific treatment methods do vary in the strength of scientific evidence for their efficacy (Chambless & Ollendick, 2001; McHugh & Barlow, 2010; Miller & Wilbourne, 2002), and people hope their health care providers are keeping up with emerging science about what works (Miller, Zweben, & Johnson, 2005). "Specific ingredients and common factors are not mutually exclusive but work together to make psychotherapy effective" (Wampold & Ulvenes, 2019, p. 69).

In this book, we focus primarily on what providers contribute to counseling and psychotherapy. We chose this focus because it is so often overlooked, and because you can do something about it. You can actually *improve* your own therapeutic competencies in relating with your clients (see Chapter 12). At the very least, you can avoid doing harm, but the positive opportunities for helping people change are much greater. The weight of evidence is clear: Both what you do and how you do it as a helper make a difference, sometimes a large difference, in the well-being of your clients.

So, what is it that more effective therapists do? That is the focus of Part II.

KEY POINTS

- Seven decades of research show important and often large differences among therapists in client outcomes even when delivering the same highly structured treatment.
- These therapist differences are consistently related to therapeutic interpersonal skills, not to therapists' age, years of experience, personality, or theoretical orientation.
- Some therapists with low levels of therapeutic skills actually harm their clients, rather than merely being ineffective.
- Helping professions have a responsibility to weed out or retrain those who are likely to provide services that change people for the worse.
- The expression of therapeutic skills varies between, and also within, therapists' own caseloads.
- Not only are overall therapeutic skills important, but also your ability to adapt how you use those skills with clients who vary in many ways.
- It matters both *what* you do and *how* you do it.

PART II

THERAPEUTIC SKILLS

In this volume, we focus on what makes a better service *provider*; that is, the impact of professional helpers themselves. If therapist factors contribute more to outcome than do the specific treatment procedures being used, what accounts for those differences? Why do providers vary so widely in their clients' outcomes even when they are ostensibly delivering the same manual-guided evidence-based treatment? Though recognizing the usefulness of recipes and ingredients, we are interested here in developing better chefs. Whatever specific treatment methods you happen to use, we are writing here about *how* you do what you do.

Chapters 3–10 describe eight therapeutic skills of more effective therapists:

- Accurate empathy
- Acceptance
- Positive regard
- Genuineness
- Focus
- Hope and expectation
- Evoking
- Offering information and advice

In each chapter, we begin with a description and some background on the skill itself. Next, we describe the therapeutic attitude behind the skill—its internal experiential aspect. Then, we turn to its external expression: how it looks in practice. Finally, we summarize what is known from research about this skill and its relationship to treatment outcome. Chapter 11 draws together the eight therapeutic skills, examining commonalities and whether there may be a higher-order "way of being" behind them.

CHAPTER 3

Accurate Empathy

"Empathy" is a word that has many meanings. We begin with a brief consideration of empathy as a trait that is part of normal human development. We then describe the therapeutic skill of accurate empathy, and explore its underlying attitude and interpersonal expression. Finally, we summarize a long history of research linking therapist empathy to better client outcomes across various forms of counseling and psychotherapy.

Trait Empathy

The experience of empathy is highly evolved in humans (Hojat, 2007) and includes at least two separate but related components with distinct neuroanatomical foundations. The first of these is cognitive perspective-taking: reading the apparent inner experience and intention of others amid complex and sometimes conflicting cues (Fonagy, Gergely, & Jurist, 2002; Lamm, Batson, & Decety, 2007). It is easy to imagine how this ability could convey an advantage within small bands of evolving humans who needed to cooperate and understand each other in order to survive. This ability to anticipate others' intentions can bestow a competitive advantage in sports, debate, games, or conflict.

A second component of trait empathy is shared affective responding: to recognize and experience, at least in part, another person's emotion. Particular types of neurons "mirror" the actions and emotions of others (Gallese, Gernsbacher, Heyes, Hickok, & Iacoboni, 2011), observable in changes in heart rate and electrical skin conductance (Critchley, 2009). An example is feeling sadness or fear during a movie. Particularly relevant for present purposes, these changes can be concordant between speaker and listener. The physiological responses of a therapeutic dyad can become empathically entrained during treatment sessions (Levenson & Ruef, 1992; Messina et al., 2013). Co-feeling can occur in counseling and psychotherapy, with the therapist not only recognizing, but partially experiencing a feeling such as sadness or joy that a client is expressing.

Shared affective responding may inspire compassionate action, but can also evoke responses that are not in the best interest of the individuals involved or of society. Paul Bloom (2016) cautioned against impulsive responding to affective empathy and instead advocated "rational compassion"—objective humane decision-making—to avoid biases generated by sympathy. A classic example is whether to move a particular child up the waiting list for organ donation, based on emotional empathy (Batson, Klein, Highberger, & Shaw, 1995).

Trait empathy is partially heritable (Hojat, 2007) and probably normally distributed in a population (Gillberg, 1996). Individuals may be unusually high or low in empathy, with most being somewhere in between. Some people seem to have a keen natural talent for understanding what other people are thinking, feeling, and meaning. Others may enhance their skill by various means. As with other talents like musical ability or athletic prowess, empathy can be increased by life experience (Fox, 2017; Miller & C'de Baca, 2001) or intentional practice (Miller, 2018; Thwaites et al., 2017). The practice of therapy itself may increase clinicians' capacity for empathy.

The Skill of Accurate Empathy

Within the context of helping relationships, "empathy" has a particular meaning. It is a skill more than just a trait or inner experience. It is not the same as sympathy, feeling sorry *for* someone. The skill of accurate empathy does not require feeling the same thing another person is feeling at the same time she or he is experiencing it. Co-feeling may happen, but even if it does, that in itself is not particularly help-ful to the other person. In fact, therapists often moderate their own expressed affect to counterbalance clients' emotional arousal (Soma et al., 2020). Nor is it necessary for you to have had similar experi-ence yourself in the past. In fact, if your own experience causes you to *identify* with the person, it can actually interfere with accurate empathy. Having similar experience now or in the past is neither nec-essary nor sufficient for you to provide accurate empathy. Finally, it is not just perspective-taking (the capacity to put yourself in another's position and imagine what she or he may be experiencing), although that is a *prerequisite* for accurate empathy.

A central aspect of this skill is seeking to understand the client's own perspective and experience. Therapists low in this skill appear to pay little or no attention to the client's perspective. Those with high skill in accurate empathy show a deep understanding of a client's meaning, typically talking less than the client does and reflecting their understanding back to the client (Perez-Rosas, Wu, Resnicow, & Mihalcea, 2019). Accurate empathy is both an observable skill (as described below) and an internal experience or attitude.

The Attitude of Accurate Empathy

A starting point is knowing that each person has experience that is, in some ways, like all other people's, like some other people's, and like no other person's (Kluckhohn & Murray, 1953). You have enough in common with your clients to be able to grasp some of their meaning and experience, and yet it is wise to have a beginner's mind and not assume that you understand fully. A fundamental attitude in empathic understanding is *curiosity,* an openness to and interest in another's experience. Often curiosity about human experience is what attracts people to helping professions. A wonderful aspect of being human is that you are not limited to your own experience and perspectives. With flexible openness, you know that you do not start with an accurate understanding of another person's life, and you *want* to understand (Lazarus, Atzil-Slonim, Bar-Kalifa, Hasson-Ohayon, & Rafaeli, 2019). You're willing to take the time to enter into the client's frame of reference, to look through the lens with which he or she perceives the world.

In ordinary conversation, people tend to listen just long enough to reply. With accurate empathy, you listen with the intent to *understand*. You set aside, at least for the time being, the expression of your own perspectives and wisdom. Your whole attention is focused on understanding what *this* person is experiencing. The intensity of concentration and absorption is akin to the discipline of mindfulness meditation (S. C. Hayes, Lafollette, & Linehan, 2011; Kabat-Zinn, 2016; Thich Nhat Hanh, 2015).

> *Each person has experience that is like all other people's, like some other people's, and like no other person's.*

There is an unfolding quality to empathic listening. Starting with a beginner's mind, you gain gradually deeper levels of understanding of the person's meaning and experience. Listening in this way involves a continuing openness that resists the premature closure of telling yourself (or your client), "OK, now I've got it."

Your internal experience of empathy is of little use to your client unless you communicate it. As will become apparent below, this ongoing process of reflecting back your understanding also makes your understanding deeper and more accurate. By offering your empathic reflections and listening carefully to your client, you come successively closer to accurate understanding.

The *How* of Communicating Accurate Empathy

A helping relationship involves understanding and appreciating another's experience, being able to perceive reality from his or her perspective *as if* you were that person. Yet, something is still missing if you only have these *internal* experiences of empathy. Accurate empathy is a therapeutic skill, a particular kind of outward expression of understanding (Gelso & Perez-Rojas, 2017). It involves conveying your internal understanding to your client.

It is easy to *misunderstand* someone's meaning and experience. What you imagine or assume that someone is thinking or feeling can be inaccurate. How, then, can you develop the skill of *accurate* empathy? That is the focus of the rest of this chapter.

> *Accurate empathy involves conveying your internal understanding to your client.*

Three Ways Communication Goes Wrong

Behind what someone says to you is an unspoken meaning to be conveyed, and there are at least three ways in which you may misunderstand that meaning. First, people don't always say exactly what they mean. The words a client speaks convey only part of what she or he means. What is said, and how it is said, might be colored by the speaker's motivation to please, to create a good impression, or to deceive. Furthermore, the same words can have widely varied meanings to different people or in particular contexts. Meaning is also conveyed by the "music" of speech: tone of voice, pace, volume, and pauses that give more information beyond the words that would appear on a transcript.

A second place where communication can falter (besides people not saying what they mean) is through mishearing. Did you correctly hear the words that were spoken? Mishearing might happen due to inattention, background noise, accents, hearing impairment, or listening in a language that is not your native tongue.

Even if you do get the words completely right, there is a third potential source of misunderstanding, which is your own *interpretation* of what they mean. When you hear a word, you essentially look it up in your mental dictionary and consider the possible meanings, perhaps choosing the one that seems most likely to be correct. This all happens instantaneously, automatically, and often unconsciously. The danger is in assuming that your interpretation of the words you think you heard is what the person actually meant.

Silence

One way of listening is to keep silent, to say nothing in response to what you hear. Indeed, there is value in allowing people time to process what they are saying. Counselors do well to develop a tolerance for silence, resisting the urge to say something after a few seconds' pause in conversation. Yet, too much silence can leave a speaker wondering what the listener is thinking, and it invites people to project their imaginings onto the listener. This was an intentional strategy in classic psychoanalysis, using therapist silence to elicit and study clients' projections. Unless you want to invite projections, however, it is better not to be unresponsive for long spans of time. In ordinary conversation, speakers take turns inserting their personal perspectives and reactions. In helping relationships, though, the focus is on the client's well-being, and it is usually unhelpful for counselors to be regularly inserting their own perspectives, opinions, advice, and agreement or disagreement as might occur in ordinary conversation. In accurate empathy, the therapist's responses convey emerging understanding of what the client means and is experiencing.

Roadblocks to Listening Well

Accurate empathy is, in part, defined by what you are *not* doing while listening. Thomas Gordon (1970) described 12 kinds of responses that people often offer instead of good listening. He characterized these as *roadblocks* in that speakers are easily diverted by them and must, in essence, go around them in order to keep on exploring their original train of thought and experience. These responses can literally get in the way of empathic listening. Here in paraphrase are Gordon's 12 roadblocks to listening, beginning with those that counselors may be more likely to offer:

1. **Probing** is asking questions to gather facts or obtain more information.
2. **Advising** includes making suggestions and providing solutions.
3. **Reassuring** includes comforting, sympathizing, or consoling.
4. **Agreeing** is telling people they are right, perhaps approving or praising them.
5. **Directing** is telling a client what to do, as if giving an order or a command.
6. **Persuading** can be lecturing, arguing, disagreeing, giving reasons, or trying to convince logically.
7. **Analyzing** offers a reinterpretation or explanation of what someone is saying or doing.
8. **Warning** involves pointing out the risks or dangers of what a person is doing.
9. **Distracting** tries to draw people's attention away from what they are experiencing, as by humoring or changing the subject.
10. **Moralizing** is telling people what they should do and why they should do it.

11. **Judging** can take the form of blaming, criticizing, or simply disagreeing.
12. **Shaming** can have a demeaning or ridiculing tone, or apply a disapproving label.

We hasten to add that there are times when some of these responses are appropriate in helping relationships. It's just that they are all different from empathic listening and tend to divert the person away from what he or she is saying or experiencing. Agreeing, for example, can communicate that the listener has heard enough and no more needs to be said. This may be helpful if you want to move forward, but much less so when the goal is to deepen your understanding of a client's experience. Asking a question requests information about some particular aspect of what the person was saying, potentially derailing the original direction of self-exploration. It's not wrong to agree or to ask a question. It's just different from (and often easier than) accurate empathy.

Empathic Listening

What is accurate empathy? It is a way of listening that helps you avoid roadblocks and step inside another person's world. It is not passive, but *active* listening (Gordon, 1970; Gordon & Edwards, 1997; Miller, 2018), a kind of mirroring. You give your full attention to what the person is saying, and you also *reflect back* your understanding. James Finley (2020) described a psychotherapist as "someone who keeps inviting you to slow down and listen at the feeling level to what you just said." It's not an echo chamber in which you merely repeat what you heard. Rather, you make a guess about what it means, what has not (yet) been said. Instead of merely reiterating a client's words, you speak what might be the *next* sentence in the paragraph. At first, you may stay closer to the person's words, but as you gain understanding, you make gradual guesses (Miller, 2018; Nichols, 2009).

SPEAKER: It's been a pretty rough week.

LISTENER: You've been having a hard time.

SPEAKER: I'll say! Nothing seems to be going right.

LISTENER: Not the way you hoped.

SPEAKER: I guess I'm not surprised, really, but our daughter's been spending time again with friends we told her she shouldn't see anymore. She just doesn't listen.

LISTENER: You're pretty worried about her.

SPEAKER: Worried? She wound up in the emergency room the night before last.

LISTENER: You're more than worried!

SPEAKER: We just don't know what to do. I feel like we've tried everything to get her on the right track, but she's not thinking about her future. It's like she doesn't care.

LISTENER: You *do* care, though, and aren't willing to give up on her.

SPEAKER: I just feel so helpless sometimes.

Notice how, with small changes, this might be one continuous paragraph:

> "It's been a pretty tough week. I've been having a hard time. Nothing seems to be going right, not the way I hoped. I guess I'm not surprised, really, but our daughter's been spending time again with friends we told her she shouldn't see anymore. She just doesn't listen, and I'm pretty worried about her. More than worried. She wound up in the emergency room the night before last. We just don't know what to do. I feel like we've tried everything to get her on the right track, but she's not thinking about her future. It's like she doesn't care. I do care, though, and I'm not willing to give up on her. I just feel so helpless sometimes.

Such mirroring allows people to stay focused on, and take a closer look at, their own experience. It also allows you to confirm (or correct) your understanding of what the client is trying to say, and conveys that you care about what he or she is saying.

Notice that the reflections above are statements, not questions. Aware that you are making a guess, there can be a tendency to inflect your voice upward at the end, which turns it into a question. That has an unintended effect of questioning (rather than understanding) what the client has said. The result can be that the client backs away from what was said rather than continuing to explore it. For example, can you see how these pairs of reflections might yield different responses?

"You're feeling anxious?" *or* "You're feeling anxious."
"You're angry with her?" *or* "You're angry with her."
"You don't see anything wrong with what you did?" *or*
"You don't see anything wrong with what you did."

The difference can be subtle, but reflections as statements tend to flow like a normal conversation, whereas the same words posed as questions may foster defensiveness.

What to Reflect?

How do you decide which aspects of clients' statements are important to reflect? The act of reflection focuses on particular facets of what someone says, selectively emphasizing or strengthening them. No one reflects randomly; to do so would be bizarre. In listening to clients, therapists make implicit and often unconscious decisions about what is important to highlight.

Of all the things clients say, a counselor "must be able to separate the wheat from the chaff" (Truax & Carkhuff, 1967, p. 160), but what is the wheat, the most important content to reflect? These are moment-to-moment decisions in any conversation, and there have been various proposals:

- A common belief is that a person's underlying feeling or emotion is particularly important to reflect (Gordon, 1970).
- Charles Truax and Robert Carkhuff (1967) suggested that the "most reliable" clue of what is therapeutically meaningful is "outward signs of upsetness, anxiety, defensiveness, or resistance" (p. 291), and recommended selectively reinforcing three themes: (1) human relationship, (2) self-exploration, and (3) positive self-concept.
- Leslie Greenberg and Robert Elliott (1997) proposed that therapists should reflect the client's experiences, particularly those of intense vulnerability, so that they can be brought more fully into the moment (p. 183).

Some authors have suggested that what is reflected, and indeed how much empathy is expressed, should be aligned with the needs of the client. Certain clients may be less able to tolerate expressions of empathy and prefer a more "businesslike" therapist (Elliott, Bohart, Watson, & Greenberg, 2011b). For such clients, a skilled therapist might, because of empathic understanding, actually reduce expressions of empathy.

In any event, *it matters what you choose to reflect.* An empathic listening response places particular emphasis on something a client has said, and tends to encourage more of the same. Chapter 9 will offer some examples of how differential reflection can affect client outcomes.

> *It matters what you choose to reflect.*

Overshooting and Undershooting

A subtle but important aspect of empathic listening has to do with the intensity of a reflection. Some authors have emphasized exact matching of the client's own intensity (Truax & Carkhuff, 1967), but there can be strategic reasons to modestly "overshoot" or "undershoot" expressed emotion or opinion (Miller & Rollnick, 2013). Understating often allows people to reaffirm and continue exploring what they have said, whereas overstating may prompt them to back away from what they expressed. Consider three possible therapist responses (undershooting, matching, or overshooting) to this client statement: "I'm just upset with my mother. She makes me so angry sometimes."

1. "You're a bit annoyed with your mother."
2. "You're angry with your mother."
3. "You're furious with your mother."

A client might respond quite differently to these three reflections; perhaps:

1. "Annoyed? No, I'm more than annoyed. I'm really cross with her!"
2. "Well, I don't know. She just frustrates me sometimes."
3. "Oh, it's not that bad. I know she's under a lot of stress, too."

Or, suppose a client says, "My son just keeps making the wrong choices!"

1. "You're a little discouraged."
2. "He hasn't been making good choices."
3. "He never makes good decisions."

What you choose to reflect makes a difference. If you want people to continue self-exploration of their experience, it's generally better to reflect at or a bit below their intensity level. On the other hand, an amplified reflection (like the #3 responses above) may help a client to reconsider an extreme position or overgeneralization, but only if spoken with no hint of sarcasm or criticism in the tone of your voice (Miller & Rollnick, 2013).

Research on Accurate Empathy

Of all the therapeutic factors that have been studied, accurate empathy has the most consistent relationship to positive client outcomes. In a meta-analysis of 82 independent samples representing more than 6,000 clients, empathy showed a moderately strong relationship with client outcomes ($d = 0.58$, $p < 0.001$) across a wide range of theoretical orientations and presenting problems (Elliott, Bohart, Watson, & Greenberg, 2011a; Elliott, Bohart, Watson, & Murphy, 2018). Higher therapist levels of accurate empathy have predicted better outcomes in client-centered counseling (Truax & Carkhuff, 1976), psychotherapy (Elliott et al., 2011a, 2011b), cognitive-behavior therapy (Burns & Nolen-Hoeksma, 1992; Miller & Baca, 1983; Miller et al., 1980; Moyers, Houck, et al., 2016), emotion-focused therapy (Watson, McMullen, Rodrigues & Prosser, 2020), health promotion (R. G. Campbell & Babrow, 2004), motivational interviewing (Fischer & Moyers, 2014), and even computer-delivered brief intervention (J. D. Ellis et al., 2017). Empathic therapists are more likely to establish the kind of strong working alliance that predicts better outcomes (McClintock, Anderson, Patterson, & Wing, 2018). Outside the psychotherapeutic realm, empathy is strongly associated with medical patients' satisfaction with their physician, independent of factors such as waiting time or visit duration (Kortlever, Ottenhoff,

Vagner, Ring, & Reichel, 2019). Even small increases in the level of empathy of emergency room physicians can lower patients' thoughts of litigation (D. D. Smith et al., 2016).

Therapists with *low* levels of empathy in practice may be of particular concern (Mohr, 1995; Moyers & Miller, 2013). Analyses of therapist effects sometimes reveal a few therapists with outstandingly *poor* client outcomes (McLellan, Woody, Luborsky, & Goehl, 1988; Project MATCH Research Group, 1998). Poor outcomes, in turn, have been linked to therapists with low levels of accurate empathy and of Rogers's core therapeutic skills more generally (Lafferty, Beutler, & Crago, 1989; Miller et al., 1980; Valle, 1981). Truax and Carkhuff (1967) found no outcome differences between clients whose therapists had moderate or high levels of core skills, but both groups had much better outcomes than did clients whose therapists had low levels of interpersonal skills.

Do Clients Cause Therapist Empathy?

One rival explanation is that better-prognosis clients (e.g., those who are more "motivated") inspire counselors to be more empathic, and that's why therapist empathy predicts better outcomes. Empathic responding does vary within as well as between therapists. In some ways, this makes intuitive sense: Clients who are able and willing to express more of what they are experiencing offer therapists many more opportunities for expression of empathy (Barrett-Lennard, 1981). Therapists, on average, tend to show higher levels of empathy with clients who are more intelligent and show less pathology (Elliott et al., 2018; Kiesler, Klein, Mathieu, & Schoeninger, 1967). A negative therapist attitude toward a client has been linked to judgments of greater disturbance and poorer prognosis, with a potentially deleterious impact on the course of therapy (Strupp, 1960). There is also evidence that empathy levels are higher depending on the similarity between client and therapist (Duan & Hill, 1996). In contrast, Truax and Carkhuff (1967) found that therapists' core therapeutic skills (including empathy) were relatively independent of clients. Furthermore, they demonstrated experimentally that when therapists switched between high and low levels of therapeutic skill within sessions, clients' levels of self-exploration tracked the therapists' responses as predicted (Truax & Carkhuff, 1965).

The truth is likely both: that therapists do differ in their accurate empathy skills, and clients also influence the process. In sum, therapeutic empathy is co-created, with therapists having greater responsibility for their own contribution.

KEY POINTS

- Accurate empathy is a reliably measurable and learnable therapist skill that is associated with better client outcomes across a range of interventions and problem areas.

- Empathic (reflective, active) listening is a particular way of responding that mirrors a client's experience while avoiding "roadblocks."

- A skillful reflection does not merely repeat what a client says but makes a gentle guess about what may be unsaid.

- Meta-analyses indicate that empathic listening is associated with greater client self-exploration and better treatment outcomes.

- Client self-exploration can be affected by the intensity of offered reflections (undershooting, matching, overshooting).

CHAPTER 4

Acceptance

Nonjudgmental acceptance has long been recognized as an important therapeutic skill in counseling and psychotherapy, and is even regarded by some to be the most important (Wilkins, 2000). Here is an early description:

> It involves as much feeling of acceptance for the client's expression of negative, "bad," painful, fearful, defensive, abnormal feelings as for his expression of "good," positive, mature, confident, social feelings, as much acceptance of ways in which he is inconsistent as of ways in which he is consistent. (Rogers, 1957, p. 98)

In this sense, the counselor's manner is "unconditional." Clients are not required to meet certain criteria in order to be accepted or respected by the counselor. Acceptance is "the ability to listen without preconception, prejudgment, or condemnation" (Strupp, 1960, p. 99). This can be quite a departure from everyday social discourse in which people may argue, disapprove, warn, judge, analyze, moralize, criticize, blame, or express sarcasm—virtually all of the roadblocks described in Chapter 3. This very contrast with ordinary communications may be what renders acceptance so therapeutic.

In this chapter, we focus in particular on this interpersonal quality of nonjudgmental acceptance. We recognize that the term "acceptance" has also been applied to other therapeutic conditions including warmth, positive regard, and affirmation (Farber & Doolin, 2011b; Orlinsky & Howard, 1986; Rogers, 1951). In Chapter 5, we will turn our attention to these related therapeutic attributes.

The Attitude of Acceptance

Nonjudgmental acceptance is a key element in the practice of mindfulness, which gained prominence in psychotherapy research early in the 21st century, particularly in third-generation cognitive-behavior therapies (S. C. Hayes, 2004; S. C. Hayes et al., 2011), stress management (Kabat-Zinn, 2013; S. L. Shapiro, Astin, Bishop, & Cordova, 2005), and addiction treatment (Witkiewitz, Bowen, Douglas, & Hsu, 2013; Witkiewitz, Lustyk, & Bowen, 2013; Witkiewitz & Marlatt, 2004). Based on ancient contemplative practices (Anonymous, 1957; Salzberg, 1995; The Dalai Lama & Hopkins, 2017), mindfulness involves attentive observation of one's immediate experience without needing to judge or evaluate, approve or disapprove. It is an accepting appreciation of what is, without critique or demand for what ought to be.

Implicit in this therapeutic attitude is a belief that human beings have inherent worth and deserve respect without needing to earn it. This belief is not just a broad reverence for humankind, but a respect for and acceptance of this particular, unique individual, the client in front of you. Therapists seek to communicate acceptance of clients as they are, affirming their sense of inherent worth (Farber & Doolin, 2011a).

How is the expression of acceptance therapeutic? Carl Rogers's (1951) perspective was that when people experience themselves as unacceptable, they are immobilized and unable to change. Like punishment, a sense of unacceptability may suppress behavior, but it does not foster a new way of being. Paradoxically, it is when people experience unconditional acceptance of themselves *as they are*—be it from parents, a loved one, a therapist, or from God—that they are enabled to change. This runs contrary to a belief that people will change if they can just feel *bad* enough about themselves. In Rogers's view it is the very experience of unacceptability, of *conditional* worth, that causes people to reject experience that does not conform to their conditions of worth. Conversely it is the experience of nonjudgmental acceptance that is healing, even when provided briefly as by a therapist (Miller, 2000; Rogers, 1961). (An added benefit of developing this skill is that through practicing unconditional acceptance of others, you may come to more fully accept and integrate your own experience as well.) The counselor seeks to understand clearly the client's experience and reflect back that understanding, responding without judgment, accepting what the client offers. Through this modeling, clients may come to accept and respect their own experience.

Do you find yourself objecting, "Doesn't this just give people permission to do whatever they please?" In truth, people already have this freedom of choice, and further rejection or disapproval is unlikely to be remedial. Implicit in nonjudgmental acceptance is a recognition "of their right as a self-determining individual not to change, to be 'cured' or to grow" (Wilkins, 2000, p. 27). Acceptance offers the *possibility* of change.

> *Acceptance offers the possibility of change.*

Underlying Beliefs about Human Nature

Beyond a general reverence for the value of each individual, there are broader beliefs about human nature. Consider these three contrasting views about people's inherent nature (Miller, 2017; Rogers, 1962):

> *Theory A:* People are fundamentally self-serving; without social controls, they would revert to an instinctual nature that is self-centered, hostile, antisocial, and destructive.
>
> *Theory B:* People have no basic nature, but are a happenstance product of their genes and experience; they are essentially a blank slate written upon by nature and nurture.
>
> *Theory C:* People's natural predisposition is collaborative, constructive, and trustworthy; at least when given the supportive conditions for change, people will typically move in a positive and pro-social direction.

One cannot conclusively prove the truth of any of these three views of human nature, but there is evidence regarding the *consequences* of embracing one or another of these views. In management theory, Douglas McGregor (2006) differentiated what he called

"Theories X and Y." Theory X is that workers are inherently lazy and unmotivated, dislike working, and will get away with doing as little as possible. Managers who accept Theory X therefore tend to be vigilant, skeptical, and mistrustful of their employees and rely heavily on threat, coercion, restrictive supervision, rewards, and punishment to make workers do what they would otherwise avoid doing. Theory Y, in contrast, is the view that workers have untapped talents and creativity, often enjoy their work, and are capable of self-control and self-direction. It is the Theory Y manager's job, then, to provide such workers with the proper atmosphere to bring out their responsibility, motivation, and creative engagement in the workplace. Both views, it turns out, tend to be self-fulfilling prophecies (Jones, 1981), and successful businesses discovered long ago the advantages of a Theory Y organization to inspire collaborative productivity, creativity, and commitment (Deming, 2000). After all, which manager would you rather have?

There are obvious parallels in counseling and psychotherapy. The finding of significant differences among therapists is far from new. In one of the earliest studies of psychotherapists, Hans Strupp (1960) distinguished two kinds of therapists. Group I therapists were warmer, more accepting, humane, permissive, and democratic, whereas those in Group II were more directive, disciplinarian, moralistic, cold, and harsh. Therapists in Group I viewed client prognosis more optimistically; those in Group II were more pessimistic. As we will discuss in Chapter 8, perceived prognosis matters and tends to produce outcomes consistent with expectations. In another early study, John Whitehorn and Barbara Betz (1954) found that the improvement rates of clients with schizophrenia varied from 0 to 100% depending on the therapist who treated them, in a population where the average improvement rate was 50.6%. Working backward from treatment outcomes, they compared the characteristics of seven psychiatrists who had the highest rates of symptomatic improvement (averaging 75%) with those of another seven who had the lowest success rates (averaging 26.9%), even though their clients' characteristics differed only slightly. A key difference between these two groups of therapists was that the former were rated as more accepting—"respectful, sympathetic, and active"—whereas the latter were characterized as "superficial, impersonal, and passive." More recent evidence on the specific impact of therapist acceptance is reviewed below.

Resistance

The phenomenon of "resistance" is another way in which one's attitude about human nature can become self-confirming. There was once a widespread belief among clinicians working in addiction treatment that people with substance use disorders (then called "alcoholics" and "addicts") are pathological liars, extremely resistant to treatment, and characterologically dependent on immature defense mechanisms like denial. Indeed, addictions were classified as personality disorders prior to DSM-III (American Psychiatric Association, 1980). This description puzzled us because it did not match how we experienced the people we were treating. There *never was* scientific evidence that people with substance use disorders have a defining personality structure or overuse particular defense mechanisms. Addiction is not confined to particular demographics or personality types. How, then, did this view of clients' characteristic similarities become so widespread among treatment professionals? It was, in essence, a self-fulfilling prophecy. The directive, non-accepting, and confrontational style of communication that was prevalent in addiction treatment at the time naturally evokes defensiveness rather than honesty, and is thereby counter-therapeutic, fostering a pessimistic view of clients' prognosis (White & Miller, 2007). The very concept of "resistance" attributes to client pathology what is inherently an interpersonal phenomenon that is highly responsive to therapist behavior (Miller & Rollnick, 2013; Patterson & Chamberlain, 1994; Patterson & Forgatch, 1985).

In contrast, an accepting style of communication normally diminishes defensiveness. Client "resistance" can be turned up and down like the volume control of a radio by changes in therapists' response style (Glynn & Moyers, 2010; Patterson & Forgatch, 1985), and defensive or resistant client responses, in turn, predict poorer treatment outcome. Counseling in a manner that evokes resistance is unlikely to yield benefit; counseling in a way that reduces defensiveness is more likely to yield positive change.

This phenomenon may have long evolutionary roots in interpersonal communication dynamics. "Psychological reactance" refers to a well-documented tendency for people to act contrary to uninvited persuasion and advice, even if they agree with it (Brehm & Brehm, 1981; Rains, 2013; Steindl, Jonas, Sittenthaler, Traut-Mattausch, & Greenberg, 2015). Dominance hierarchies are clearly observable in higher mammals, and are governed by complex social behavior that allows the loser in a conflict to escape by signaling acquiescence (de Almeida Neto, 2017). For humans, dominance dynamics are encoded in language (often judgmental) and may operate unconsciously. Within this perspective, to comply with persuasion or advice is to accept a "one-down" position. Behavioral advice is an ideal context for triggering reactance and noncompliance, because people ultimately have discretion over their own behavior (de Almeida Neto, 2017). Consider this dialogue around behavioral activation with a client who is depressed:

> THERAPIST: I think what you need to do is to get out of the house and do some things that you enjoy around other people.
>
> CLIENT: I just don't have the energy.
>
> THERAPIST: Your lack of energy is just part of your depression, and it's not going to get any better if you stay at home with the blinds closed. You should be doing things that you enjoy.
>
> CLIENT: But I don't even enjoy things I used to like.
>
> THERAPIST: That's part of depression, too. It's called anhedonia, lack of pleasure. If you just get out and try things you used to like doing, you might find there is still some enjoyment in them.
>
> CLIENT: I doubt it.
>
> THERAPIST: Well, that's what I'm going to assign you to do this week as homework. On at least three days this week, plan to get out of the house and do something you might enjoy. You're not required to enjoy it—just do it!
>
> CLIENT: I guess I can try.

The therapist's intention is good. The advice is sound and evidence-based. In the process of this dialogue, however, the therapist takes an expert stance by persuading, advising, educating, and directing, which can feel perfectly natural to a helping professional. However, the teach/direct dynamic of this conversation is one that normally evokes defensive responses, which, in turn, predict nonadherence and lack of change (Miller & Rollnick, 2013; Patterson & Forgatch, 1985). The therapist is not listening well (Chapter 3) and not communicating acceptance.

The *How* of Communicating Acceptance

So, how does one manifest a therapeutic condition of acceptance? To an important extent, acceptance is communicated by what you do *not* do. It involves refraining from judgmental responses such as disapproving, criticizing, disagreeing, labeling, warning, or shaming. Many of the communication roadblocks that we described in Chapter 3 have the effect of placing clients in a one-down position. Even approval can be judgmental, in that it implies an appraisal (in this case, positive) of a client's experience.

"Confronting" is a therapist response with particular potential for communicating judgment and triggering reactance or resistance. The essence of confrontation can be to direct, persuade, disagree with, correct, disapprove, judge, or shame—all communication roadblocks. One observational system for therapist behavior describes a confront response as "directly and unambiguously disagreeing, arguing, correcting, shaming, blaming, criticizing, labeling, warning, moralizing, ridiculing, or questioning the client's honesty" (Moyers, Rowell, Manuel, Ernst, & Houck, 2016). A relatively small number of confront responses can undermine an otherwise productive counseling session.

How might the above dialogue be different if the therapist began with listening and acceptance?

THERAPIST: I have an idea that has worked for some other people I've seen. I don't know whether it will make sense to you, but I wonder if it's OK to tell you about it.

The therapist immediately communicates acceptance by giving the client permission to disagree ("I don't know whether it will make sense to you") and asking permission first, rather than charging into advice.

CLIENT: Sure.

THERAPIST: Part of the trap of depression is in becoming isolated from people, places, and things that you care about. Do you know what I mean?

Respectfully checking in to see if the client is following.

CLIENT: Yeah, I mostly stay at home, and I know that's not good.

Change talk (see Chapter 9) rather than resistance.

THERAPIST: And one way out of the trap is to get out and do some things that you used to enjoy, even and especially when you don't feel like it. Now, that may sound impossible to you.

Acknowledging potential reluctance.

CLIENT: No, I can see what you mean, but I just feel so tired most of the time.

THERAPIST: Of course you do; I understand. When you're feeling that tired, it's hard to imagine getting out to do anything that might be fun. It really *is* like a trap.

There is a compassionate, accepting tone here. Reflective listening in itself communicates acceptance.

CLIENT: That's right. I feel like I'm stuck and need to get unstuck.

THERAPIST: I don't know what you're willing to do, and it's up to you. I wonder, though, if you might be willing to try something new this week.

Acknowledging and honoring the client's autonomy. Asking in a way that emphasizes the client's choice.

Notice that there is still some psychoeducation happening, but in a more collaborative rather than directive way, acknowledging the truth: that clients get to decide what they will accept and do.

The etymology of *confront* is "to come face to face," and in this sense, it could be thought of not as therapist behavior ("getting *in* someone's face") but rather as a *goal* of counseling: to help clients take a close look at themselves in a safe and supportive environment. Some gentle confronting may promote self-exploration and change, but *only* in the context of a trusting, empathic, accepting therapeutic relationship (S. C. Anderson, 1968; Moyers, Miller, & Hendrickson, 2005). Communicating acceptance diminishes defensiveness and makes it safer to consider what is potentially threatening or difficult.

The absence of judgment can be surprising to clients, particularly in contexts where they have been coerced into treatment and expect harshness, like students summoned into the principal's office. Clients can be particularly sensitive to perceived blame or disapproval. Couples who come for relationship counseling may expect or fear that the therapist will decide which of them is more at fault. Feeling blamed or shamed is a recipe for defensiveness and the status quo. When clients offer vulnerable content without receiving judgment, disapproval, or immediate direction, they often are surprised and relieved.

One way to refrain from overt judgment is to keep quiet, but silence is not inherently free of judgment. The problem, as mentioned in Chapter 3, is that people may project into your silence their own worst fears and imaginings. Rather than remaining distant and silent, actively communicate acceptance in a way that reassures clients and averts imagined judgment.

One good way to communicate acceptance is through the skill of accurate empathy as described in Chapter 3. Working hard to understand someone's meaning implies respect, and is quite different from the common conversational style of listening just long enough to interject a reply, often a roadblock. Here, the underlying *attitude* of acceptance matters, because disapproval can creep into reflections just through voice tone. A mindful attitude of curiosity without judgment tunes the music behind reflective listening. Acceptance is a context within which empathic understanding can be communicated.

Actively communicate acceptance in a way that reassures clients and averts imagined judgment.

Mindfulness practices are ancient and have been incorporated in a wide range of modern therapeutic methods (Benson & Klipper, 2000; S. C. Hayes et al., 2011; Kabat-Zinn, 2016; Thich Nhat Hanh, 2015; Witkiewitz et al., 2014). Various forms of meditation involve centering of attention (e.g., on breath, a stationary object, or a mantra) while observing and accepting one's experience without judgment. If you want to help clients learn such practices as coping skills, it is advisable to be a practitioner of the method yourself. Beyond the integrity of "practice what you teach," developing the discipline of mindful meditation may offer benefits for you as well. Practicing mindful acceptance as a state can generalize and promote trait mindfulness (Kiken, Garland, Bluth, Palsson, & Gaylord, 2015).

Counseling itself can be done within a state of mindful acceptance, and the discipline of practice may help to foster acceptance as a normal response to what you experience. In this way, acceptance can become a default way of being rather than a skill to be called out as needed.

Beyond empathic listening and mindfulness, another concrete way to communicate acceptance is through the practice of affirmation, to which we will return in Chapter 5. Affirmations are direct statements of regard and appreciation for a client's positive attributes and actions. In this chapter, we focus primarily on the more general therapeutic stance of nonjudgmental acceptance, though of course it is the therapist's communication of this attitude that matters most (Horvath, 2000).

Research on Therapeutic Acceptance

There is an immense scientific literature on the benevolent effects of meditative and mindfulness practices themselves (Gotink et al., 2015; Keng, Smoski, & Robins, 2011). Our focus here is on the effects of therapist acceptance on client outcomes.

In extensive reviews of the relationship between therapist acceptance and client outcomes, David Orlinsky, Klaus Grawe, and Barbara Parks (1994) found that 56% of 154 effects were positive; still higher (65%) when therapist attributes were judged from the client's perspective. When therapist acceptance was rated independently from recordings by nonparticipant observers, and client outcome was judged from objective measures, 62% of findings showed a positive relationship (Orlinsky & Howard, 1986). Positive outcomes were also high when therapist and client were mutually accepting (79% of findings).

An interesting observation was a trend that the positive impact of acceptance increased with the proportion of racial/ethnic minorities in the sample (Orlinsky et al., 1994). This parallels a meta-analytic finding that the effect size of motivational interviewing, a person-centered therapeutic style, was tripled (d = 0.79 vs. 0.26) in samples predominantly from racial-ethnic minority groups, relative to nonminority samples (Hettema, Steele, & Miller, 2005). In both reviews, therapists in the studies were primarily nonminority. It may be that an accepting, empathic style is even more important with marginalized clients who are less accustomed to such treatment, and when counseling across significant sociocultural differences.

In sum, there is ample evidence that clients whose therapists manifest and communicate acceptance generally have better outcomes. This is just one attribute of counselors that by itself is modest in effect, but in combination with others can contribute to the large differences often observed in therapists' outcomes, even when allegedly using the same treatment techniques.

> *An accepting, empathic style may be even more important with disadvantaged clients.*

KEY POINTS

- Implicit in the therapeutic attitude of acceptance is a belief that human beings have inherent worth and deserve respect without having to earn it.

- The experience of being accepted as one is at present can facilitate positive change.

- Beliefs regarding the essential quality of human nature in general or of a particular individual can be self-fulfilling prophecies.

- Client defensiveness or resistance is an interpersonal phenomenon, and is usually diminished by an accepting, empathic, and respectful therapeutic style.

- Acceptance is communicated, in part, by what the therapist does *not* do: disapproving, criticizing, disagreeing, labeling, warning, or shaming.

- An accepting and respectful style may be even more impactful when working with marginalized groups and when counseling across significant sociocultural differences.

CHAPTER 5

Positive Regard

Warmth and respect in counseling did not originate with Carl Rogers, but he was the first to hypothesize a *causal* role for prizing clients in a sincere and meaningful way. He described "unconditional positive regard" as one of three conditions (in addition to accurate empathy and genuineness) that are necessary for healing.[1] It was a radical departure from the view that healing happens primarily through the therapist's expert knowledge and ability to execute specific technical procedures. Paul Wilkins (2000) asserted that positive regard (PR) is a "major curative factor in any approach to therapy; congruence and empathy merely provide the context in which it is credible" (p. 23).

The *unconditional* aspect of PR overlaps with our discussion of nonjudgmental acceptance in Chapter 4: that clients do not need to prove or earn a counselor's respect. PR is a precondition extended to all, without regard for apparent merit, rooted in an intentional view of humankind as inherently "positive, forward-moving, constructive, realistic, [and] trustworthy" (Rogers, 1962, p. 91; cf. Giannini, 2017; Miller, 2017).[2]

---

[1] Rogers believed empathy, genuineness, and positive regard to be not only necessary, but also *sufficient* conditions for healing to occur in counseling and psychotherapy. We do not concur that these are the only aspects of treatment that matter, though it is surprising how often these therapeutic skills are sufficient to help clients change.

[2] Though Rogers disavowed theological overtones of his work, his own graduate training did begin at Union Seminary (Kirschenbaum, 2009), and he openly explored spiritual parallels in dialogues with Martin Buber, Paul Tillich, and Reinhold Niebuhr (Kirschenbaum & Henderson, 1989).

The measurement of PR as a therapeutic attribute has had a somewhat erratic course, in part because of the number of different terms used to refer to the same or similar concepts—such as warmth, acceptance, respect, and support. Indeed, Rogers (1957) described PR as "warm acceptance" of a client's experience (p. 829). The Truax and Carkhuff (1967) scale conflated low PR with giving advice and taking responsibility for the client; whereas with high PR, the therapist showed "deep respect for the patient's worth as a person and his rights as a free individual" (p. 66).

A client self-report instrument designed to measure all three of Rogers's therapeutic conditions (Barrett-Lennard, 1962) differentiated two aspects of PR: an *overall* level of PR and the *conditionality* of that regard. The conditionality rating focused on whether the therapist's approval and warmth varied depending on what the client was expressing or doing. Thus, therapists might rate highly on their *overall* level of PR, and also show some withdrawal of that approval in response to specific content. This is of interest because Rogers clearly intended that therapists should aspire to prize their clients *regardless* of their distressing behaviors and statements. The conditionality of therapist PR proved to be less reliable and valid as a subscale, so it is often omitted in studies using the Barrett-Lennard Relationship Inventory (BLRI; Barnicot, Wampold, & Priebe, 2014). The overall PR scale has good internal consistency (= 0.91), with reasonable reliability and validity across multiple therapy process studies, and has become a gold standard in measuring therapist PR. It does not, however, specify the behaviors by which therapists can manifest PR.

The Attitude of Positive Regard

As with accurate empathy and acceptance, PR involves an experiential aspect for the therapist as well as the means for communicating it to clients. The internal experiential component of PR is a cognitive and emotional disposition, a mindset of the therapist. In the most general sense, this disposition is a stance of respect and benevolence toward your clients, a commitment to their well-being and best interests. PR is a compassionate context for the practice of all other relational elements described in this book. It would be possible, for example, to practice skillful empathic listening in order to sell a product or gain a competitive advantage. In counseling and psychotherapy, therapeutic skills are used with the intention of promoting the client's own welfare and best interests.

Rogers (1959) described unconditional PR as the therapist's attitude of "warmth, liking, respect, [and] sympathy" (p. 208). He focused on positive growth rather than pathology, an attitude also reflected in the more recent development of positive psychology that focuses on the study of human happiness, virtues, and well-being (Peterson & Seligman, 2004; Rashid & Seligman, 2018; Seligman, 2012). Rogers believed that people possess a powerful innate drive toward health and positive growth. He therefore did not regard himself to be an expert healer, but rather as a privileged witness to clients' natural ability to heal and grow even in difficult circumstances. This recognition and respect for clients' own wisdom are important components of PR.

The *How* of Communicating Positive Regard

The external aspect of PR is its behavioral expression. It is well and good to experience PR for your clients, but better still if you communicate that regard through your words and actions. PR involves treasuring and acknowledging what is positive in your clients. You anticipate and appreciate what is good within them: their strengths, accomplishments, intentions, and virtues. For demoralized clients, you perceive and convey what they do not currently see in themselves. This is a habit to cultivate, focusing on strengths and capability, and not only on problems. Here are a few examples of counselor responses that reflect PR:

- "You didn't shy away from some really difficult material today. That took some courage!"
- "As you talk about all of the troubles you've been through, do you know what strikes me? You are a real *survivor*! You've taken a lot of hard knocks, and you're still here."
- "You intended not to drink at all this week, and you had *five days* with no alcohol at all. That's amazing! How did you do it?"
- "You deeply love your children and want to do all you can to protect them."

PR statements normally begin with the word "you" rather than "I." There is something inherently evaluative when beginning with "I," even if the judgment is positive ("I'm proud of you.") Saying, "I think you're doing really well" also shifts the focus, at least partially, away from the client to you. It's better and simpler to say, "You're doing really well."

Positive regard involves prizing and acknowledging what is positive in your clients.

So, what therapist responses convey PR? The Psychotherapist Expressions of Positive Regard (PEPR) scale contains items asking clients about their therapist's verbal and nonverbal behaviors. It includes simple affirmations ("Good to see you," "That was a good session") as well as specific behaviors ("My therapist handed me a tissue when I began to cry," "My therapist encourages me to take pride in things I do well") and more general therapist attitudes reflected in multiple interactions over time ("My therapist makes a connection between my current experience and something I have done in the past," "My therapist offers me a new way of understanding a part of myself that I usually view as a weakness"). A factor analysis of the PEPR yielded two reliable factors. First, "Supportive/Caring Statements" are specific things a therapist might say to express warmth and reassurance toward a client. The second factor, "Unique Responsiveness," reflects a sense that the therapist has been deeply attentive to the client as an individual and has discovered something worthwhile in that attending. However, these two factors may simply reflect method variance in item structure, in that all items on Factor 1 are direct therapist statements, whereas Factor 2 is made up only of items beginning with "My therapist. . . . "

A third weaker factor, "Intimacy/Disclosure," contains specific items that might be viewed as boundary violations: therapist hugging, putting a hand on the client's shoulder, becoming tearful at a sad story, sharing something personal, noticing a change in the client's appearance, and getting in contact outside of counseling to check on the client after a particularly difficult session. Unlike the first two factors, this one was *negatively* related to PR as measured by the Barrett-Lennard scale.

In sum, therapists high in PR convey an overall sense of warmth, respect, and support. A separate though related concept is nonjudgmental acceptance (Chapter 4)—whether PR varies depending on what the client is expressing. Presumably, this would involve a combination of PR communications, with selective messages of disapproval or non-acceptance of particular content. Measuring therapists' PR and non-acceptance responses separately may prove more reliable than the unconditionality subscale.

Affirmation

Affirmation is a way to convey PR directly. It involves both noticing and commenting on a person's strengths, positive actions, and attributes. Affirming expresses your prizing of the person in an honest and explicit way. As with reflections (Chapter 3), it is possible to think of affirmations as either simple or complex. Simple affirmations comment on a particular behavior and may be as small as thanking a client for coming to a session, acknowledging completion of an assignment, or noticing an apparent lift in mood. Simple affirmations are relatively easy to offer and don't cost you much in cognitive or emotional effort, yet they can provide glimpses of your PR and appreciation. Being inexpensive, simple affirmations can also be overused and may appear disingenuous even if they are well intentioned. They don't speak directly to what it is about the *person* that you appreciate. As with simple reflections, relying on simple affirmations can limit depth of relationship.

Affirmation involves noticing and commenting on a person's strengths, positive actions, and attributes.

Complex affirmations involve more effort on your part. They require listening for strengths, finding what you can appreciate and admire in a client as a person. It is easy to forget this in the press of details and problems that may quickly emerge in a therapeutic encounter. Yet, we know therapists for whom genuine affirming seems to come as naturally as breathing. Perhaps you do, too. For most of us, it is a gradually acquired practice, to stay alert for and comment on what is positive even in the midst of chaos. It is an acquirable skill (Muran, Safran, Eubanks, & Gorman, 2018). In essence, complex affirmations are internal, stable (trait) attributions of something positive (Weiner, 2018). Here are some examples of complex affirmations:

- "Even though you didn't want to come here today, your love for your wife helped you to decide. It sounds like you care for her very much."
- "With all the obstacles that you've overcome, and now this

latest one, you just keep right on going. You're someone who is really determined even when the going is rough."

- "Now that's a really creative idea! You come up with solutions that might not occur to other people."
- "You're a person of your word. Once you make a commitment to someone, they know they can rely on you."

In essence, you are connecting current experience to something that is more enduring and admirable about the person. To see things from this viewpoint can help clients feel encouraged, heartened, optimistic, and willing to take risks or make difficult choices. Of course, this can happen in many kinds of relationships—with a teacher, a coach, or a friend. Being treasured and appreciated can be a profound experience.

Embedded Positive Regard

PR is also communicated in many ways besides direct verbal affirmations. Clients may value what you *do* even more than what you say about them (Suzuki & Farber, 2016). Clients can feel valued, for example, when therapists listen well or are flexible with appointments. PR is communicated, in part, through nonjudgmental acceptance (Chapter 4) and by the very act of accurate empathy, taking time to understand a person's meaning (Chapter 3). Without saying so directly, these actions convey the message, "You are someone worth listening to, and whose words matter."

Here is a connection between the internal and external aspects of PR. Therapists who hold a positive, accepting, and optimistic attitude toward clients are more likely to convey embedded, interwoven expressions of PR that go beyond direct affirmations. These emerge from your ongoing appreciation of clients' strengths, strivings, and accomplishments in the moment.

We suspect that the internal optimistic attitude of PR is not easily taught in training or through reading this book. The good news is that you can learn it from your clients. Accompanying clients on their journeys through difficult human experiences while *looking for the good in them* can afford greater appreciation of human resilience, and more capacity for PR with the next person, and the next. The discipline of looking for what is positive in the client sitting across from you is never wasted.

Can Affirming Be Harmful?

Some therapeutic traditions are wary of therapist affirmation. One expressed reason (described but not endorsed by Gelso & Kanninen, 2017) is a concern that gratifying clients' need to be appreciated may divert them from the self-examination necessary to mature beyond requiring such approval from others. By not gratifying immature and neurotic needs, the therapist hopes to help clients seek more mature ways of being. Such withholding of gratification is a common depiction of psychoanalysis, though warm and interactive analysts deplore this stereotype. Although it is conceivable that withholding affirmation might cause clients to mature, we know of no clinical science to support this, whereas there is ample evidence (reviewed at the end of this chapter) that affirmation and expressing PR are associated with better outcomes for clients. In choosing between the risk of being too withholding or too affirming, we favor the latter.

Of course, affirming can go badly. Shallow or inaccurate affirmations may backfire, coming across as empty disingenuous praise. There will also be differences in response to affirmation across clients and cultures. A client who begins treatment with mistrust of manipulation may respond warily to early affirming. The obvious caveat here, as with the other skills that we describe, is to observe carefully how your clients respond. With some clients, you may need to *earn* the opportunity to express PR through genuineness, acceptance, and empathy during a probationary period. Affirmation should be titrated depending on your clinical judgment and feedback from the client. The interpersonal norms of affirmation also vary. In some cultures and subcultures, overt expressions of warmth and appreciation are common, whereas in others they are sparse. The interpreted meaning of affirmation can vary. It might be perceived as manipulation or disguised criticism. If you do misstep in affirming, though, you are likely to find out by paying attention to your client's reaction, and can make adjustments to repair a rupture in the working alliance (Rubino, Barker, Roth, & Fearon, 2000; Safran, Crocker, McMain, & Murray, 1990). In any event, retain the internal experience of perceiving, admiring, and treasuring the strengths in your clients.

As with most therapeutic interpersonal skills, there is a Goldilocks balance in the expression of PR: neither too much nor too little for each person, but an amount that is just right. There is also a lot of skill in *how* affirming is done—for example, in leaning forward, looking a client in the eye, or speaking in a gentle voice.

Here's an illustration from an initial session with a woman who has Type 2 diabetes and has been referred to discuss health behavior and lifestyle changes. It combines empathic listening and acceptance with examples of positive regard (PR).

> CLIENT: This is all new to me. I can't quite believe that I actually have diabetes. I feel fine.
>
> THERAPIST: This really took you by surprise. You've been healthy and would like to stay that way.
>
> CLIENT: Right. I keep in pretty good shape.
>
> THERAPIST: You're *already* doing things to take good care of yourself and stay healthy! You just didn't expect this news.
>
> CLIENT: The doctor said it could be pre-diabetes instead of diabetes.
>
> THERAPIST: You're hoping it might not be so serious yet.
>
> CLIENT: I don't know. I don't want to pretend it's not serious if it is.
>
> THERAPIST: It sounds like you're open to the facts, and are considering what you can do to stay well.
>
> CLIENT: Yes, that's important to me.
>
> THERAPIST: Good for you, because you're the one who's most likely to know what will work for you in making some healthy changes.
>
> CLIENT: I've been thinking about it.
>
> THERAPIST: Already! Let me ask you this. I wonder when you have had to make a significant change in your life before. It doesn't have to be about your health—just any important challenge you've faced that required some changes from you.
>
> CLIENT: Like my divorce?
>
> THERAPIST: Exactly. How did you manage?
>
> CLIENT: I had to learn to do a lot of things on my own, things I hadn't much done before.
>
> THERAPIST: You became more independent; able to do some new things.

CLIENT: Yes, I guess I did. I had to.

THERAPIST: So, when something unexpected happens, you're a woman who figures out what to do, and how to do it.

Don't worry about figuring out which therapeutic skill corresponds to each response here. An empathic reflection can also sound like acceptance or affirmation. In this illustration, the counselor is highlighting the client's strengths, motivations, positive efforts, and freedom of choice.

Research on Positive Regard and Affirmation

Meta-analyses reflect a modest positive effect size ($g = 0.27$–0.28) of PR on treatment outcome (Farber & Doolin, 2011a; Farber, Suzuki, & Lynch, 2018). After controlling for duplicate use of datasets and study samples across the 64 included studies, the effect size in these analyses increased to a moderate level ($g = 0.36$). This is somewhat smaller than the estimated effect sizes reported for accurate empathy (Chapter 3) and genuineness (Chapter 6). In a clinical trial of depression treatment (Barnicot et al., 2014), therapist PR did not predict client outcomes, whereas genuineness and empathy did.

Why such variability? In part, the low predictiveness may be related to varying definitions of PR. Therapist affirmation is a more specific construct than PR, based on reliably observable practice behavior. Psychological research indicates that affirmation (including self-affirmation) tends to diminish defensiveness, facilitating the consideration of potentially threatening information and behavior change (Critcher, Dunning, & Armor, 2010; Epton, Harris, Kane, van Konigsbruggen, & Sheeran, 2015; W. M. P. Klein & Harris, 2010).

As with reflections (Chapter 3), it also apparently matters what content you affirm. Consistent with the principle of positive reinforcement, clients who receive therapist affirmation following a statement are more likely to continue making statements of the same kind, including maladaptive content (Karpiak & Benjamin, 2004). In the same study, therapist affirmation of "maladaptive" content in client speech predicted poorer 12-month outcomes from cognitive-behavior therapy.

In a conditional probability study, therapist affirmations were significantly *less* likely to be followed by client speech defending continued drinking (sustain talk), and more likely to be followed by client change talk (Apodaca et al., 2016). That is, affirmation preceded clients' increased interest in changing problematic behavior and decreased defense of the status quo.

It appears that PR and affirming can have a positive therapeutic influence, even in an online format. Fredrick Holländare and colleagues (2016) found that therapist behaviors of affirming and encouraging were significantly associated with client improvement during an Internet-based cognitive behavioral intervention for depression.

A noteworthy clinical trial was published by Marsha Linehan, the progenitor of dialectical behavior therapy (DBT). Women meeting diagnostic criteria for both opioid dependence and borderline personality disorder were randomly assigned to receive either DBT or a novel comparison treatment called comprehensive validation therapy (CVT) and participation in 12-step programs (Linehan et al., 2002). All clients were offered opioid maintenance and, of course, had free access to 12-step meetings. CVT contained "nondirective" components of DBT including therapist warmth and genuineness, acceptance-based strategies, and validation, but none of the directive behavioral procedures of DBT. The affirming component of CVT (and DBT) was described thus: "The therapist watches for valid responses in session or reports of valid responses out of session and responds with immediate validation" (p. 24). The authors noted that their prior efforts to apply behavior therapy had not been effective "until comprehensive validation was added to the treatment, suggesting that validation may be the key treatment factor" (p. 16). In this sense, it was a dismantling trial, testing the additive impact of specific therapeutic components beyond CVT.

The two treatments were similarly effective in reducing opiate use across 16 months of treatment and follow-up, with a small advantage for DBT during Months 8–12. There were no dropouts from CVT during a year of treatment, as compared with 36% among DBT clients. Reductions in psychopathology and parasuicidality were substantial, with no differences between groups. In sum, the full DBT program was not more effective than its affirmation/validation components.

———————— **KEY POINTS** ————————

- Along with accurate empathy and genuineness, Rogers described unconditional PR as one of three necessary therapeutic conditions to facilitate positive change.

- The experiential (internal) aspect of PR for therapists is an unconditional respectful and benevolent disposition toward clients, anticipating and appreciating their strengths and potential for growth.

- The external aspect of PR involves its behavioral expression in practice, communicating PR to your clients.

- Affirmation is a reliably observable practice behavior associated with lower defensiveness and better therapeutic alliance and outcomes.

- Simple affirmations comment on a particular client behavior, whereas complex affirmations focus on clients' positive strengths and traits.

CHAPTER 6

Genuineness

Some professional helpers are expected to remain objective, personally removed, opaque, and unbiased by subjective emotional responses. Judges, for example, are not generally expected to be spontaneous, emotional, transparent, or funny. The same might be said of dentists or detectives, nor does transparency befit a professional poker player. In some lines of work, especially when personal contact is sporadic or scarce, taking work seriously means mostly keeping aspects of the genuine self away from human exchanges. This distance lends an objectivity that is needed for the tasks at hand. Personal relationships are non-essential to the work and can even be a distraction.

For other professions, however, genuineness is an asset. Master teachers and mentors, for example, take their work seriously, and also have a knack for bringing their humanity into it. They strike a balance. Some objectivity is essential, and there are professional boundaries to be honored; yet a lack of genuineness can compromise the working alliance that improves outcome.

As with acceptance (Chapter 4), the nature of genuineness may be clearest when it is absent. Disingenuousness involves hiding yourself in some way. Without an authentic presence, helpers may cling to a role, often as an expert or a detached observer. Partly for self-protection, they may appear to be reserved, detached, or wholly objective. In short, they keep far too much of themselves out of their professional interactions. Think of a student in a clinical training program who is seeing clients for the first time. Experiencing anxiety, lack of confidence, and "imposter syndrome" can limit genuineness, creating a stiff, artificial presence. Fortunately, most counselors grow out of the need to hide themselves, learning to bring valuable aspects of their humanity to working with clients.

Physicians illustrate this professional balance. In a health care setting, patients expect a certain degree of objectivity, competence, and confidence in their caregivers. They want a professional who keeps up with the scientific literature and will offer the advice or

> *Disingenuousness involves hiding yourself.*

treatment that is most likely to help them be well. Given a choice between a distant but competent healer and one who is kindly but incompetent, most would prefer the former. Thankfully, such a choice is unnecessary because a professional can be both competent and genuine (Gordon & Edwards, 1997). Indeed, doctors who relate and listen well tend to have patients who are more likely to follow their advice and have better health outcomes (Rakel, 2018; Rollnick, Miller, & Butler, in press).

Therapists' genuineness is greater when they spend less effort concealing themselves and instead respond in ways that are uniquely and authentically their own (Gelso & Carter, 1994). Presence, real relationship, openness, honesty, and non-phoniness are other terms that have been used to describe this characteristic of helping professionals who do not hide themselves at their clients' expense (Geller & Greenberg, 2018; Kolden, Klein, Wang, & Austin, 2011; Weinraub, 2018). Qualities of spontaneity, humor, and vulnerability promote a working alliance with clients. In practice this means being (1) aware of your own inner experiences with clients, (2) emotionally engaged as the client's story unfolds, and (3) willing to reveal your own experiences, thoughts, emotions, and values *when they benefit your client* (Schnellbacher & Leijssen, 2009). In other words, genuineness means the therapist as a person shines through, rather than being hidden behind a façade (Lietaer, 2001a).

Although genuineness has been the least studied of Carl Rogers's three therapeutic conditions, it can be measured within helping relationships and is relevant in their success (Grafanaki, 2001; Truax & Carkhuff, 1976). There are both observational rating scales and behavioral measures.

The original measure of counselor genuineness was a scale devised by Charles Truax and Robert Carkhuff (1967) based on observation of treatment sessions, usually via audiotape. As with their other rating scales for nonpossessive warmth and accurate empathy, the genuineness scale rated counselors at one of five levels or stages. At the lowest level was clear defensiveness, with obvious discrepancy between the therapist's words and experience (e.g., shouting "I am not angry!") Slightly higher genuineness (Level 2) was indicated by responding in a "professional rather than personal manner" that sounds "contrived or rehearsed." Above the midpoint, Level 4 was an absence of defensiveness (explicit or implicit) or of apparent incongruence between experience and self-report. The highest rating (Level 5) required not only a lack of defensiveness or distant professionalism, but also being very much oneself, showing congruence with one's own feelings and experiences.

The Barrett-Lennard Relationship Inventory (BLRI: Barrett-Lennard, 1962) and the Real Relationship Inventory (RRI: Kelley et al., 2010) have been the two most common methods for capturing clinician genuineness via a self-report questionnaire. The BLRI can be completed by both the therapist (self-assessment) and the client (evaluating a therapist). For example, the BLRI asks therapists to rate themselves on the following statement: "I am willing to tell (my client) my own thoughts and feelings," whereas the client's version states: "(My therapist) is willing to tell me his/her own thoughts and feelings." The RRI similarly has two versions with items focusing on behaviors of the therapist in the session (e.g., "My therapist was holding back his/her genuine self").

A behavioral measure related to genuineness is therapist self-disclosure. This will be discussed later with the communication of genuineness.

Congruence: The Inner Experience of Genuineness

Therapeutic genuineness can be understood as having both internal and external components (Kolden et al., 2011; Lietaer, 2001a, 2001b). The internal or experiential component, which we will refer to as "congruence," is a necessary but not sufficient prerequisite for the external manifestation of genuineness, which we will call "authenticity." (Note that both of these terms—congruence and authenticity—have sometimes been used as synonyms for genuineness.)

There is a direct relationship between your ability to extend acceptance to others (Chapter 4) and your self-acceptance, which, in turn, is related to congruence. If you are uncomfortable with your own experience, it is difficult for you to help others accept and integrate theirs. "When I discover that I am accepted and loved as a person, with my strengths and weaknesses, when I discover that I carry within myself a secret, the secret of my uniqueness, then I can begin to open up to others and respect their secret" (Vanier, 1998, p. 82).

Congruence is the degree of convergence between a person's self-perception and his or her actual experience. Rogers (1957) applied the concept of congruence as an indicator of mental health for both clients and psychotherapists, and for people more generally. Incongruence, a cause of suffering and pathology in Rogers's theory, involves non-acceptance of what one actually feels, thinks, or does. In this sense, incongruence parallels Carl Jung's concept of the shadow as aspects of the self that are denied or not fully conscious (Jung, 1957; Jung, Read, Adler, & Hully, 1969). Non-acceptance of your own imperfections augurs blindness to or projection of these characteristics in others. As one pithy saying goes, "You spot it, you got it." Counselor self-acceptance is regarded as necessary to experience and convey other core therapeutic conditions such as empathy and warmth (Truax & Carkhuff, 1976).

Within the context of a helping relationship, congruence also involves awareness of how clients are affecting you in real time during sessions, and an acceptance of your own feelings and impressions as they arise. Here, congruence overlaps with the psychodynamic concept of counter-transference, the therapist's own feelings and reactions to a client (Wilkins, 2000). Self-awareness of your own responses to clients is an important component of responsible practice (Burwell-Pender & Halinski, 2008; Pieterse, Lee, Ritmeester, & Collins, 2013).

Authenticity: The *How* of Communicating Genuineness

Congruence with your own experience is different from how you communicate it interpersonally, including within helping relationships. It is possible to be aware and accepting of your inner experience and still knowingly or unknowingly present a façade to clients. As an interpersonal characteristic, genuineness involves offering an authentic representation of your experiencing within *this* relationship at *this* time. Self-concealment, on the other hand, has been linked to a wide variety of adverse health outcomes (Larson, Chastain, Hoyt, & Ayzenberg, 2015).

The goal of therapeutic genuineness is not to be working through your own feelings within a session. Rather, a primary aim is to avoid deceiving yourself or your client. Authenticity is when your internal experiences can be revealed to clients in a way that facilitates a therapeutic goal. Genuineness, then, involves both congruence—recognizing and accepting your internal experience—and authenticity—accurately conveying your experience with empathy (Watson, Greenberg, & Lietaer, 1998). It is easy to imagine that clinical training might impact one of these components but not the other. The human capacity for congruence and authenticity often expands through life experiences, including personal psychotherapy.

Genuineness should always occur within the larger interpersonal context of acceptance, empathy, and positive regard. Genuineness without empathy is no gift. When clients experience your empathy, acceptance, and affirming positive regard, it can smooth potentially rough edges in honesty. Transparency should always be grounded in these larger therapeutic conditions (Watson et al., 1998). Genuineness means awareness of your own reactions to what is happening with clients, and the ability to convey them through an empathic filter in order to serve your clients' best interests.

Honesty and empathy can sometimes be conflicting values. There are times when helping professionals consciously choose *not* to say exactly what they think or feel, and this may be particularly important when clients are fragile or severely troubled. Still, counselors who are relaxed, empathic, accepting, and honest in responding are more likely to be helpful than harmful, even when working with clients who are disturbed, touchy, or contentious. A key question is this: Are you unforthcoming in order to benefit the client, or to serve your own needs?

Negative Emotions toward Clients

A common reason for clinicians to choose interpersonal distance over genuineness is the avoidance of intense negative emotion that can arise with some clients from time to time. In some ways, this is an understandable choice. Feeling frustration, disgust, or anger toward a client is not unusual (Pope & Tabachnick, 1993), and these feelings are toxic to a therapeutic relationship if not responded to wisely by the therapist (Wolf et al., 2017). So, what is an authentic therapist to do? Thankfully, the cure lies in the characteristic of genuineness.

Being able to recognize and accept your own negative feelings about your clients is a necessary first step in responding wisely. Therapists who are low in congruence will have particular difficulty recognizing and acknowledging such feelings. When you experience and acknowledge negative feelings toward a client, consider at least two important questions. First, do these feelings have something to do with your own history, personality, or values? Second, do these feelings mimic what other people may experience when interacting with this person? Answering these questions involves being both a participant and an observer in the process, which itself may relieve some of the intensity of negative emotions.

It is also wise to cultivate practices to regulate your own normal, reflexive, and potentially harmful emotions toward clients (Wolf et al., 2017). Such practices can include mindfulness (Davis & Hayes, 2011; Kelm, Womer, Walter, & Feudtner, 2014), and developing specific methods for responding to therapy-interfering behaviors (J. A. Hayes, Gelso, & Hummel, 2011) and for enhancing and repairing ruptures in the therapeutic relationship (Safran et al., 2014). As Abraham Wolf and colleagues (2017) observed, "We believe that these experiences and the ways they are dealt with in psychotherapy explain, at least in part, therapist effects—the fact that some therapists are better and, perhaps more particularly in this case, worse than others" (p. 176). As with clients, it is not the presence of negative emotions themselves, but rather how one responds to them, that can influence therapeutic outcomes.

Self-Disclosure

In terms of specific counselor responses, self-disclosure is an observable behavior logically related to genuineness. Yet even at the highest level of genuineness on the Truax and Carkhuff (1967) scale, there was no requirement for therapists to disclose their personal feelings or experience; only to avoid being dishonest, defensive, or incongruent about them. The issue of whether, when, what, and how counselors should self-disclose is an enduring question that is directly relevant to genuineness (Knox & Hill, 2003), and too often bypassed in clinical training. Opinions vary on the wisdom of self-disclosure, with some concerned that it may undermine therapists' *gravitas* and professional distance, or serve the therapist's own needs (Farber, 2006). Within a person-centered approach, professional distance and *gravitas* are undesirable, and are precisely what one does *not* want in a therapeutic relationship.

Empirical findings regarding self-disclosure are somewhat more consistent. Counselor self-disclosure has been associated with better therapeutic relationship and client outcomes (Hill, Knox, & Pinto-Coelho, 2018), particularly when disclosure reveals the therapist's humanity or similarity to the client (Henretty, Currier, Berman, & Levitt, 2014; Levitt et al., 2016; Somers, Pomerantz, Meeks, & Pawlow, 2014). In general, self-disclosing people tend to be perceived as more likable, trustworthy, and having more favorable personal characteristics (Collins & Miller, 1994).

As with many virtues, an excess of transparency can be detrimental. You are under no obligation to say everything that you think and experience, nor should you, because doing so may be hurtful. Being genuine does not mean following any impulse in thought or action as it occurs in counseling. Neither does it mean being brutally honest. Self-disclosure is appropriate *when it is likely to be helpful to the client*. Professional counselors are not co-clients, working through their own personal issues in therapy sessions. There should be a conscious reason why you believe a particular self-disclosure is likely to be beneficial, and then carefully observe the client's reaction. A theoretical model for how people change can guide you in what types of disclosures may be useful and which are better left unsaid.

> *Self-disclosure is appropriate when it is likely to be helpful to the client.*

Genuineness does mean avoiding dishonesty. A cardinal violation of genuineness is to pretend that you are not thinking or feeling something when you actually are. "Therapist commitment to truthfulness promotes client acceptance of the problems they face as well as efforts to change" (Kolden et al., 2011, p. 69). Denying what is true is dishonesty, and clients readily see through it, often due to inconsistency between your verbal and nonverbal behavior. It may be that what matters most is not a high level of genuineness, but the absence of counselor phoniness (Grafanaki, 2001).

A particular choice-point in self-disclosure comes when a client asks you a question about yourself:

- "Do you have children?"
- "Have you ever felt this way?"
- "Did you ever use drugs?"
- "Are you married?"
- "Do you drink?"
- "Where do you live?"
- "Do you find me attractive?"

The decision as to whether and what you disclose is yours to make, influenced by your comfort in providing the information and your judgment about the likely impact on the client and your relationship. To provide personal information may step across an appropriate boundary that should be maintained in psychotherapy. To refuse or be dishonest may impair your working alliance. Professional dispositions vary between "always disclose" and "never disclose," with most therapists found somewhere in between these extremes, depending on the content.

It is appropriate to consider why the client may be asking this question. In our university training clinic, clients occasionally ask a young therapist, "How old are you?" Sometimes it is possible to guess the motivation that underlies a client's question, and one possible starting point is to reflect his or her concern.

CLIENT: How old are you?

THERAPIST: You're wondering whether I have enough experience to help you.

CLIENT: Well, yes. You look so young. So much younger.

THERAPIST: And, of course, that concerns you! You took a big step in coming here; I can see that you are heavy-hearted, and you want to work with someone who can understand and help you.

CLIENT: Yes, I do.

THERAPIST: Let me tell you a little about how we work here, and then you can let me know if you're comfortable working with me. OK? [Honoring autonomy]

CLIENT: OK.

THERAPIST: This is a training clinic, just as our university hospital is a training hospital. The therapists are in doctoral-level training, and we have completed most of our coursework. Here in the clinic, we are closely supervised by faculty who are licensed psychologists, and who meet with us weekly to ensure the quality of our work. Is that what you understood?

CLIENT: Yes, the man on the phone told me you would be in training.

THERAPIST: I promise to listen to you well, to understand your concerns, and work together toward the changes you hope for. I will do my best to help you, and am comfortable that I can, but it is important for you to be comfortable as well. What do you think?

CLIENT: I'm willing to give it a try.

In this particular case, the therapist did not answer the initial question but addressed the underlying concern. It's also possible to provide an answer, but don't overlook why the client is asking. Here is how we respond to a common question that comes up in addiction treatment:

CLIENT: Have you ever used drugs? Are you in recovery?

THERAPIST: I will tell you the truth, but before I do, there are two things I would like to know: What will it mean to you if my answer is "yes," and what will it mean to you if my answer is "no"? So first, what if I *have* used drugs and am in recovery?

CLIENT: I guess mostly I'd feel like you might be able to understand me better, and not judge me.

THERAPIST: Fair enough. You want to work with someone who can understand you, and won't be judgmental about what you say.

CLIENT: Right.

THERAPIST: OK. Anything else before we talk about the other side?

CLIENT: If you got out of *the life* yourself, I guess I'd be interested in how you did it.

THERAPIST: Great! You're open to ideas for your own recovery. Now what would it mean to you if my answer is "no"?

CLIENT: Well, I guess I'd wonder if you can really help me then. I'm not sure I should listen to somebody who's not in recovery.

THERAPIST: Understandable. Again, you definitely want a counselor who can understand you, won't be judging you, and can help you.

CLIENT: Right. So, what is it?

THERAPIST: When I was young, I did drink more than was good for me, and I also tried some drugs a few times. I quit the drugs, though, and I drink very little now. I'm not in recovery from addiction myself.

CLIENT: Why are you here, then?

THERAPIST: Because I'm clear that this is where I can make a life-and-death difference, and because I keep seeing so many people get so much better. May I tell you something that might interest you?

CLIENT: Sure

THERAPIST: Studies consistently show that people's treatment outcomes are just as good whether or not their counselor is in recovery. I understand that you might feel more comfortable if I had experience just like yours, but I've been working with people here for 19 years, and I would enjoy working with you. I hope that I can.

CLIENT: I just thought that you could tell me about recovery.

THERAPIST: And I can. You don't have to listen to what I tell you. It will be up to you to take what's useful and leave the rest. But I do promise that I will listen to you!

Research on Genuineness

Though therapists are not unanimous regarding the value of genuineness, results from meta-analyses have been reasonably consistent across the decades, indicating that like counselor self-disclosure, genuineness improves working alliance and treatment outcome (Gelso, Kivlighan, & Markin, 2018). Citing 10 prior reviews, Gregory Kolden and colleagues (2011) concluded that "empirical support for the contribution of congruence to client outcome is mixed, but leaning toward a positive endorsement" (p. 67). A subsequent meta-analysis of 21 studies relating counselor congruence to client outcomes documented a moderate estimated effect size of d = 0.46 (Kolden, Wang, Austin, Chang, & Klein, 2018).

As with research on other therapeutic conditions, client reports of therapist genuineness tend be more reliable than therapist self-reports when predicting observer ratings of in-session therapist genuineness. Furthermore, clients' ratings of therapist genuineness predict treatment outcome, whereas therapist self-ratings often do not (Gelso et al., 2012). This in itself is an interesting observation on genuineness!

Relationships among therapeutic conditions are also informative (Gelso & Carter, 1994). Client BLRI session ratings were studied in a large multisite trial for the treatment of depression (Barnicot, Wampold, & Priebe, 2014). All three core conditions (empathy, genuineness, and unconditional positive regard) were rated separately to tease apart their individual associations with outcomes as measured by the Beck Depression Inventory (BDI). Clinician genuineness was associated with lower depression during treatment and also modestly predicted decreased depression *after* treatment, regardless of the initial severity of the depression.

Research indicates that the relationship between ratings of therapeutic conditions and client improvements is accounted for by true differences among clinicians, and not simply because some clients elicit favorable reactions from therapists whereas others do not (Baldwin, Wampold, & Imel, 2007; Barnicot et al., 2014; Zuroff et al., 2010). Therapist skills such as genuineness can also account for unique variance beyond that related to working alliance (Coco, Gullo, Prestano, & Gelso, 2011). Together, these findings make a respectable case that a clinician's ability to convey genuineness can improve treatment outcomes.

Open questions about genuineness remain. Less scientific attention has been devoted to genuineness than to other therapist characteristics such as empathy, and many published studies have been based on analog experiments rather than actual therapy sessions

(Grafanaki, 2001). Additional research on this topic could advance not only the clinical science of psychotherapy but also an understanding of other human exchanges in which genuineness plays an important role. Relatively little is known, for example, about how genuineness develops and how it might be strengthened in clinical training and supervision (Lietaer, 2001b).

As with all of the therapeutic practices we describe, there will be individual differences in how clients respond. Nearly all research on genuineness has come from Western nations, and there may be cultures, subcultures, or contexts within which it would be more effective for therapists to adopt a more authoritative and less "authentic" role. It is also possible that genuineness or "real relationship" may be the most important of a therapist's interpersonal skills, without which empathy and acceptance have little meaning for the client (Greenberg & Geller, 2001; Lietaer, 2001b). After all, what value do therapist empathy and acceptance offer to a client who perceives them to be disingenuous? Genuineness, we believe, is worth further exploration, both with individual therapists and in the helping professions more generally.

KEY POINTS

- Although distant objectivity is regarded as important in some professions, it appears that therapists who are warm, open, and honest tend to have better client outcomes ($d = 0.46$) and working alliance.

- Rather than high levels of genuineness per se, it may be a lack of phoniness and dishonesty that matters in counseling and psychotherapy. In fact, an excess of transparency can be detrimental.

- Genuineness should always occur within the larger interpersonal context of acceptance, empathy, and positive regard.

- Congruence, the intrapsychic component of genuineness, is a necessary but not sufficient prerequisite for its external manifestation as authenticity.

- Genuineness can be reliably measured by both Likert rating scales and the observation of specific therapist responses, both of which have been linked to better client outcomes.

CHAPTER 7

Focus

In a frequent paraphrase from Lewis Carroll, "If you don't know where you're going, any road can take you there"; or in Yogi Berra's rendition, "If you don't know where you're going, you might wind up somewhere else." A long-acknowledged characteristic of more effective therapists is that they have clear goals and a coherent plan for reaching them with their clients (Beutler, Machado, & Neufeldt, 1994; Frank & Frank, 1993; Imel & Wampold, 2008). As with affirmation (Chapter 5), there is a matter of balance here, in that too tight a focus can be detrimental. Think of a spotlight highlighting an actor. Too tight a beam could illuminate just one part of the person, perhaps a foot. Too broad a beam floods the whole stage or auditorium, and focus on the actor is lost. When working with clients who are ambivalent or reluctant about change, premature tight focus can damage therapeutic alliance. A guiding balance is needed to maintain both therapeutic direction and empathic connection with clients (Miller & Rollnick, 2013).

With each new client, an initial step for focusing is to clarify the goals of your work together. "A specific goal or subgoal in the therapeutic situation tends to accelerate the progress" (Truax & Carkhuff, 1967, p. 361). Having common goals shared by therapist and client is a key component of a good working alliance, which, in turn, predicts better treatment outcomes (Flückiger et al., in press; Horvath, Del Re, Flückiger, & Symonds, 2011; Horvath & Greenberg, 1994; Tryon & Winograd, 2011). Clients may cherish and be willing to pay for the companionship of a sympathetic listener (Schofield, 1964), but without clear goals, outcomes are amorphous, and sessions may continue indefinitely. In our view, it is not responsible or desirable for therapy to continue indefinitely, wandering without direction. Many agencies require a treatment plan that specifies objectives and the intended means to reach them, which encourages accountability in the therapeutic process. Governmental and other third-party payers for behavioral health services likewise favor evidence-based treatment shown to produce particular outcomes. How could one know whether a treatment is effective without knowing what it is intended to effect?

Having a clear focus is by no means universal in practice. In ongoing counseling, a surprising amount of time can be used in informal "chat" that may be unrelated to clients' treatment needs (Martino, Ball, Nich, Frankforter, & Carroll, 2009). One study found that higher levels of such off-topic chat were linked to lower client motivation for change and retention in treatment (Bamatter et al., 2010).

The Attitude of Focus

One element of focus in therapeutic relationships is a felt responsibility to have a clear direction for your services: a shared understanding of the goals of your work with each client, and an organized plan for reaching those goals. What would constitute a positive outcome with this client? In certain contexts, such as a smoking cessation clinic, the intended outcome is well defined. With other contexts and clients, the goal(s) of counseling may be less clear at the outset, and a formulation process is needed to determine a consensus direction. If you find yourself wandering through several sessions without a shared understanding of goals, a soft warning light should be flashing. An inner experience of focus is a sense of discomfort, if for session after session you have no identified goals for your work together. It's fine for goals to change over time; that's common in counseling and psychotherapy. Clarity of focus is knowing where you want to go together, and having a provisional plan for how to get there.

Clarifying and maintaining focus is an important professional responsibility, usually reflected in a treatment plan. Part of the attitude of focus is maintaining continuity of direction over time.

Particularly in a busy practice, this can require checking your treatment plan and notes prior to each session, to remember what progress has been made thus far with a particular client and to identify what a next step might be. Without such continuity, it is easy to just respond to crises and whatever topic a client raises. Some clients may want

Clarity of focus is knowing where you want to go, and having a provisional plan for how to get there.

to update you in each session on whatever is happening in their lives, like catching up with a friend.

Again, there is a balance involved. Finding and maintaining direction in treatment should not occur at the expense of accurate empathy, acceptance, positive regard, and genuineness. These therapeutic skills provide an interpersonal context for continuity of focus.

The *How* of Focusing

Who determines the goal(s) of treatment? Ideally, this happens through a process of negotiation, and there are at least three potential sources of treatment goals: (1) your client, (2) the context, and (3) you as a provider. Clients typically present for treatment with specific concerns in mind that they want to address, and in one sense a treatment goal is not a goal—certainly not a shared goal—until the client concurs with it. (We discuss conflicting treatment goals later in this chapter.) A further consideration is that your actual "client" may, at least in part, be a referring agent with particular goals (Monahan, 1980), as in cases like these:

- Someone court-mandated to treatment after a drunk driving or domestic violence offense
- An adolescent brought in by parents for treatment of behavioral problems
- A physician's patient referred for help in better managing diabetes
- A supervisor referral to an employee assistance program

It is also the case that treatment goals may be shaped by the service or context within which you work. When a client comes through the door of a weight loss clinic, there is little ambiguity about the primary topic of conversation. Some settings specialize in relationship enhancement, addiction treatment, anxiety or depression, domestic violence, or pain management. Some contexts limit the outcomes that are acceptable. Historically, some addiction programs would treat only clients who accepted a goal of total abstinence from certain (or all) psychoactive drugs. Specific pregnancy counseling centers may be unwilling to support a client in choosing an abortion. Such context-driven limitations can tighten the focus, and can also pose significant dilemmas in supporting client autonomy and self-determination (Ryan & Deci, 2017).

There are also times when you, as a provider, perceive priorities other than those initially presented by a client. One such scenario is when you suspect an underlying cause for the problems that prompt a visit. For example, a physician may perceive that repeated visits for medical concerns are related to a patient's drinking or smoking. A mood or stress disorder might be linked to relationship problems. Sometimes you may, in the course of consultation, simply detect another clinical issue that in your opinion ought to be addressed, even if it is unrelated to the presenting problems. Here, the challenge is raising a potential change that was not among the client's presenting concerns.

The focusing process, then, is one of finding direction for treatment among these various and sometimes conflicting potential goals. This involves shared decision-making (Barry & Edgman-Levitan, 2012; Elwyn & Frosch, 2016). Sometimes the goal is reasonably clear at the outset: for example, a man recovering from a

Focusing involves finding direction for treatment among sometimes conflicting potential goals.

heart attack who wants to stop smoking, or a distressed couple seeking help to improve their relationship to which both are committed.

In other cases, focusing involves choosing and prioritizing among a variety of options for change, a process that Stephen Rollnick termed "agenda setting" (Rollnick, Miller, & Butler, 2008). In diabetes management, for instance, there are many possible paths toward better glucose control and health promotion (Steinberg & Miller, 2015). Figure 7.1 shows a sample "bubble sheet" that a health psychologist or diabetes educator might use to introduce possibilities for health behavior change.

"Here are a dozen different things that people can do to get better control of their diabetes and prevent complications in the long run. Some of these steps you may already be taking. I wonder if there are one or two here that you might like to talk about today. Or, perhaps there's something even more important that you want to discuss. That's why there's a blank bubble. Which of these do you think might be a good place to start?

Then there are times when specific directions for change aren't clear at all. This can happen, for example, following a major upheaval—a divorce, job loss, or death of a loved one. The structure

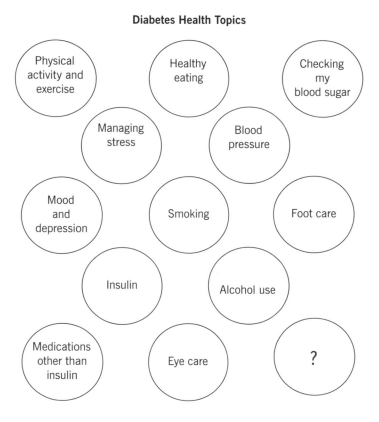

Diabetes Health Topics

FIGURE 7.1. A sample "bubble sheet" for diabetes health topics. From Steinberg and Miller (2015, p. 17). Copyright © 2015 The Guilford Press. Reprinted by permission.

and meaning that had previously served as an organizing container for life are suddenly shattered. Such major and abrupt change can leave people in disarray, deeply distressed, and confused. In other cases, it just seems like *everything* is wrong, and it's unclear where to start or what is beneath it all. After an initial period of good empathic listening, you begin together formulating possible directions for change.

Resolving Ambivalence

Sometimes establishing a consensus focus with a client can be challenging, even when the problem seems clear and straightforward. It is not that the problem is hidden or complex, but rather that the client is ambivalent about changing it. People are often ambivalent when contemplating difficult changes. Reluctance about change is quite normal, even when clients are presenting for treatment and asking you to help them change. If you fail to recognize and address this ambivalence, it may worsen as you attempt to implement change procedures such as giving advice, recommending ways to alleviate distress, giving between-session practice assignments, or explaining the cause of the client's problem. A familiar response when you tell someone what to do, how to do it, and why it's important is, "Yes, but . . . " This is sometimes viewed as resistance or denial, but it's actually a predictable result of your defending one side of a person's ambivalence (Engle & Arkowitz, 2006; Miller & Rollnick, 2013). The more you persuade and argue for change, the more likely a client will argue against it (Miller, Benefield, &Tonigan, 1993); and in turn, the more a client verbalizes reasons against change, the less likely change will occur (M. Magill et al., 2018). A common mistake in counseling and in relationships more generally is to pursue focused problem-solving when someone is ambivalent and needs good listening.

When you encounter this kind of ambivalence, you have arrived at an important choice point in how to proceed. One option is for you to maintain neutrality, sometimes called "equipoise." In this case, you carefully avoid even inadvertently nudging clients in any particular direction. Instead, you do your best to help clients reach a decision with which they are at peace (Janis & Mann, 1977). Indeed, making a choice can itself be a focus. Neutrality is an important option for situations in which you believe you should avoid influencing a particular decision or direction; for example, whether to donate a kidney to a relative. In medical care, this is referred to as *shared decision-making,* denoting situations in which physicians perceive more than one legitimate course of action (Elwyn et al., 2014). The goal in shared decision-making is to arrive at a decision, rather than promoting a particular course of action that may be favorable to the provider. Some psychotherapists regard neutrality as their *only* appropriate professional stance with any client issue. We will have more to say about neutrality later in this chapter.

A more common clinical situation is that you want to help clients move past ambivalence toward a specific goal–most often because that is what they have asked you to do. How, then, can you help clients resolve ambivalence when change is the goal? For one thing, you can pay careful attention to clients' language as they speak about their dilemma (see Chapter 9). Movement toward change is associated with more client "change talk" (stated motivations and advantages for change) than "sustain talk" favoring the status quo (Baer et al., 2008; S. D. Campbell, Adamson, & Carter, 2010; Moyers et al., 2007; Vader, Walters, Prabhu, Houck, & Field, 2010). The clinical style of motivational interviewing (Miller & Rollnick, 2013) has been shown to influence this balance of change talk and sustain talk, which mediates subsequent behavior change (M. Magill, 2018; Moyers, Houck, Glynn, Hallgren, & Manual, 2017; Moyers & Martin, 2006; Moyers, Martin, Houck, Christopher, & Tonigan, 2009). By responding carefully and preferentially to clients' language, you may influence the direction in which they move. In essence, you are helping your clients talk *themselves* into changing (Miller & Rollnick, 2004).

Sometimes getting over the hump of ambivalence is all that's necessary, after which your client may need little else from you. For example, once your client has decided to make a change, he or she may be quite clear how to go about it. Other times resolving ambivalence about change is just the beginning of progress, and other clinical skills may be needed from you to help clients implement the changes they have decided to make.

There are some situations that prescribe a certain focus or treatment goal regardless of clients' ambivalence. If you're a probation officer, for example, you're probably not doing your job unless you are encouraging your supervisees to move away from criminal behavior, even if they are not initially on board with this goal. Similarly, therapist indifference about change is unlikely if you treat people convicted of sex offenses or driving while intoxicated. To be sure, there are ethical issues in deciding what is in a client's "best interest" (Koocher & Keith-Spiegel, 2016; Miller, 1994), but it is common for treatment providers to have a preferred direction of change in mind.

Counseling with Neutrality

What if you do choose to remain neutral? How can you proceed if you want to be careful *not* to influence a client's direction of choice or change? When should you maintain neutrality and consciously refrain from directional influence? This is an ethical consideration, the resolution of which is usually not provided by therapeutic methods themselves. Discussion of therapeutic neutrality is too often bypassed in clinical training. Theories of personality may contain assertions about what constitutes a good life, but decisions about neutrality usually are a matter of clinical judgment, whether consciously or unconsciously.

Neutrality may not even be an issue if there is already a clear goal for change. The goal might be what your client has asked you to help with, and you concur. Sometimes it is a matter of urgency. When staffing a suicide prevention hotline, counselors rarely intend to be neutral about whether callers will kill themselves. Similarly, when clients are engaging in life-threatening behavior, such as injection drug use or high-risk sexual behavior, therapists are unlikely to be neutral about the preferred direction for change.

In other cases, the issue being presented by a client may be one on which you choose to remain neutral, and consciously avoid nudging people in one direction or another. Nevertheless, because you do choose what questions to ask, what content to reflect, what to affirm, and what to include in summaries, you may be inadvertently influencing clients to move in a particular direction. Remaining truly neutral can be more challenging than it may seem. This is at least partly because your own values and expertise are likely to bias the questions, affirmations, and reflections that you offer.

It is important, first of all, to be conscious of your clinical intention. Are you pursuing a clear direction for change, or do you choose to maintain neutrality? In either case, you would show equanimity and supportive professionalism. Neutrality is not a counselor attribute, but a conscious clinical decision to try *not* to influence a specific client's direction of choice or change. The counselor's decision remains in each clinical situation:

> "Should I proceed strategically to favor the resolution of the client's situation in a particular direction?"

or

> "Do I choose to maintain neutrality and *not* intentionally or inadvertently steer the person in one particular direction?"

In the latter case, the focus is to help clients reach a carefully considered decision with which they are at peace, without yourself influencing the direction of choice. A client might be trying to decide whether to adopt a child, to develop a will, to leave or stay in a job or relationship. When you want to help with the decision-making process and also want to remain neutral, how

Are you pursuing a clear direction for change, or do you choose to maintain neutrality?

can you best do that? How can you "first, do no harm" even inadvertently?

A helpful framework for vigilant decision-making was introduced by Irving Janis and Leon Mann (1976, 1977). In modern usage, their approach is often reduced to a "decisional balance" containing four cells. The original method was considerably more complex, but a four-cell structure can serve to illustrate it.

Imagine a client (individual or couple) struggling with the decision of whether to have a child. The biological clock is ticking, and the time to decide is growing shorter. If you chose neutrality as your clinical stance, how might you proceed? For a binary choice, the factors involved could be represented as follows:

	Having a child	Not having a child
The good things (pros, advantages)	A	B
Less good things (cons, disadvantages)	C	D

If you were favoring change in a particular direction (Miller & Rollnick, 2004), you would pay more attention to the cells on one diagonal. Differentially asking open questions about, reflecting, affirming, and summarizing material from Cells A and D would favor deciding to have a child, whereas selectively evoking material from Cells B and C would favor deciding to not have a child. Maintaining a balance of neutrality requires vigilance in exploring *equally* all four cells. This involves conscious effort. It would be natural enough to ask about one cell (advantages of having a child) and continue reflecting and affirming what you hear, then drawing it together by summarizing all of the client's arguments for being a parent. Here is how it might happen:

THERAPIST: There must be some things that appeal to you about having a child now. Tell me about those.

CLIENT: Having children seems like such a special experience, to give life to a new human being. I think it's a unique kind of relationship to be a parent; not one you can have in any other way.

THERAPIST: You don't want to miss out on having that kind of relationship.

CLIENT: Right! And we have to decide soon. I guess adoption is also an option, but I'm curious what our own children would be like.

THERAPIST: You can imagine what they might be like.

CLIENT: I do. You never know exactly, of course, but I know we would love them however they are.

THERAPIST: That kind of loving is important to you.

CLIENT: I want us to experience it, and I'm afraid that if we pass up the chance, we could regret it for the rest of our lives.

THERAPIST: That sounds lonely.

CLIENT: Or empty, maybe. Something like that.

THERAPIST: So, having a child or children could open up a whole new experience for you, a new dimension to your life together.

CLIENT: I think so.

THERAPIST: What might you enjoy most about it?

CLIENT: The baby years look great. When I hold an infant, it's a wonderful feeling, and I think it must be so much deeper when it's your own child.

THERAPIST: A very special kind of relationship. What else?

CLIENT: Watching them grow, discovering the world. I would look forward to each new step, to be with them as they have each new experience.

THERAPIST: You already have a sense of wonder about that.

CLIENT: I do! There must be nothing like it.

THERAPIST: So, what you've told me so far is that you think there is something unique, special about a parent–child relationship, something that you couldn't have any other way. You would treasure the baby years, and also anticipate being there as your child grows up and encounters each new step in development. You look forward to experiencing the special kind of love that parents show for their children, and I sense that it could expand your own relationship, your own world.

The therapist's responses are strong in accurate empathy, and this conversation could continue along this line for quite a while. What neither therapist nor client may realize is that they are differentially focusing on motivations for having a child, even if this was not what the counselor intended. It happened by asking an open question that focused on Cell A on page 74, and then following with good empathic listening.

Counseling with neutrality entails asking with equal curiosity about each of the four cells on page 74, listening well to and remembering what the client offers, and helping draw together a balanced summary of the pros and cons of each alternative for the client.

Of course, it's possible that there are more than four cells in the illustration. In the current example, adoption might be considered as a third option. A brainstorming process could further expand the range of alternatives. Discussion might reveal underlying and potentially conflicting values. Counseling with neutrality requires patient and balanced exploration of the alternatives, to help your client reach a considered decision that will persist with minimal post-decisional regret (Janis, 1959; Janis & Mann, 1976).

It is also worth noting that if your goal is to move toward a particular change, there are good reasons *not* to construct a decisional balance that gives equal emphasis to pros and cons (Nenkov & Gollwitzer, 2012). A decisional balance intervention with clients who are still ambivalent has been found to *decrease* commitment to change and increase commitment to the status quo (Krigel et al., 2017; Miller & Rose, 2015). Why would this be the case? If one succeeds in equally eliciting from clients their arguments for and against change, the expected outcome would be ambivalence, which in transtheoretical terms is associated with *contemplation* rather than *preparation* and *action* (Prochaska et al., 1994; Schumann et al., 2005).

When Goals Conflict

It happens, of course, that at times a client's treatment goals conflict with those of the provider or program. Perhaps the least desirable therapeutic situation is an adversarial relationship, where the provider's goal is to *make* a client change, which naturally evokes the client's complementary role of psychological reactance, defending personal freedom and resisting change (Beutler, Harwood, Michelson, Song, & Holman, 2011; Brehm & Brehm, 1981; Karno & Longabaugh, 2005). Even *advising* change can elicit such reactance (de Almeida Neto, 2017).

It also matters how *invested* you are in a particular outcome. Therapists who are too detached from client outcomes may provide insufficient focus or direction, and appear impersonal or uninterested. At the other extreme, too high a personal investment in a particular outcome can result in a desire to "carry the client across the finish line" no matter what. This is likely to evoke reactance and resistance. There is something of a sweet spot in the middle, where you are interested in working toward positive outcomes, and also honor clients' autonomy to make their own choices (Ryan & Deci, 2017).

Especially in contexts where clients might expect an adversarial relationship (such as probation or mandated treatment), give priority to developing a collaborative working alliance as a vital first step. Engagement is particularly important when you do not have shared goals at the outset. Therapeutic processes like accurate empathy (Chapter 3), acceptance (Chapter 4), and affirmation (Chapter 5) can help to forge a working alliance before developing a shared focus, let alone a plan for change. William Miller and Stephen Rollnick (2013) have described a sequence of therapeutic processes from engaging (developing a trusting therapeutic relationship), to focusing, to evoking motivation for change, and finally to planning. Jumping straight into planning, particularly when treatment is mandated or clients are ambivalent for other reasons, is unlikely to foster positive change.

Particularly in situations where clients feel pressured to change, recognizing and honoring their autonomy are not only therapeutic, but also an acknowledgment of the truth. Even under conditions of extreme control, people still exercise self-determination and make decisions (Frankl, 2006). Despite (and sometimes because of) our best efforts to direct the behavior of clients, offenders, or our own children, people do make their own choices. Human beings may be willing to pay a heavy price rather than make changes that others want for them. To tell people that they *can't* do something (drink, smoke, or leave the city) is not only inaccurate, but can also promote the forbidden. Efforts to enforce external control can even undermine autonomous motivation for change. Emphasizing personal choice may decrease the need to defend the status quo and can facilitate autonomous motivation for change (Deci, Koestner, & Ryan, 1999; Deci & Ryan, 2008; Ryan & Deci, 2008). Accepting and affirming your clients' autonomy to make choices represent a powerful therapeutic stance, and one that can be genuine and empathic as well. With Carl Rogers (1962), we believe that people, when given the supportive conditions for change, naturally tend to move in a positive, pro-social, self-determining, and healthy direction. At least *part* of them wants to do so. That part of their ambivalence is your co-therapist.

Research on Focus

A broader context for therapeutic focus is the substantial psychological research literature on goal-setting (Bandura, 1986; Ford, 1992; Locke & Latham, 1990). Meta-analyses have clearly established that setting an achievable goal promotes change, particularly when accompanied by feedback about goal attainment (Mento, Steel, & Karren, 1987; Neubert, 1998; Tubbs, 1986; Wood, Mento, & Locke, 1987). The same is found to be true in the context of psychotherapy, where goal-setting facilitates achievement of treatment goals (e.g., Swoboda, Miller, & Wills, 2017). In particular, therapist–client consensus on goals predicts better outcomes (Tryon & Winograd, 2011). This goal-consensus effect is often seen as supporting power-sharing and a collaborative working relationship with clients, with which we concur. Such consensus is not possible, of course, unless goals of therapy are present, specified, and mutually accepted.

When the goals of therapy are agreed upon, progress is much more likely. Conversely, when therapy does not focus on goals that brought the client to treatment, it is less likely to be helpful (Wampold & Imel, 2015).

Clinical research also sheds some light on what happens when focus is lacking. Illustrative in this regard are studies in which a bona fide psychotherapy is compared with a control treatment that is intended to be *like* therapy, but without the active ingredients of the preferred approach. Often, these control treatments intentionally have little structure, coherent rationale, or guiding theory for the therapist to follow (Wampold, 2015). In such comparisons, a robust difference typically emerges: The bona fide treatment with a clear focus is more effective. As discussed in Chapter 8, this could also be attributable to therapist expectancies.

Bruce Wampold (2015) has more generally discussed the need for a clear, coherent rationale as a therapeutic factor contributing to the effectiveness of therapies regardless of their specific content. This is not to say that "anything goes." As discussed in Chapter 2, specific treatment methods and therapeutic skills can have independent or interacting effects on treatment outcome. Indeed, it is implausible that it makes no difference what one does in counseling and psychotherapy. Our emphasis in this chapter is that regardless of treatment approach, it is helpful to have consensual goals and a plan for moving toward them.

────────────── **KEY POINTS** ──────────────

- Focusing is a shared decision-making process to identify clear goals for consultation.

- Client outcomes are generally better when counselors have clear treatment goals and an organized approach to achieve them.

- Ambivalence about change is normal, and helping to resolve it is an important therapeutic process.

- Advising, persuading, or pushing clients toward change tends to elicit psychological reactance and to diminish the likelihood of change.

- Neutrality is a conscious decision in a particular clinical situation where the client is ambivalent, and decisional balance is a helpful tool to avoid inadvertently influencing the client's direction of choice.

CHAPTER 8

Hope

Does your own optimism about your clients' potential to succeed have any impact on their outcomes? Do clients find strength and encouragement to pursue change from your own positive expectations? What if you are feeling pessimistic or burned out by your work: Is there a remedy? As you might guess, we believe the answer to all of these questions is "yes," and we hope that by the end of this chapter, you will agree.

Let's begin with one of our favorite pieces of research about hopefulness. Three different inpatient treatment programs agreed to participate in a study of alcoholism recovery using a specially designed personality test. The researchers identified clients whose scores on the test indicated particularly high alcoholism recovery potential (with the clients referred to as HARPs) and shared the assessment results with the program counselors. To protect confidentiality, counselors were asked not to share these test results with anyone else.

The test performed admirably. Although the HARPs were no different from their peers on common prognostic factors such as problem severity and prior treatment history, they differed in other important ways. None of the HARPs left treatment prematurely, whereas one-third of other clients did so. When clients were asked to rate each other, their peers described HARPs as more desirable to be with and showing better recovery. Counselors also rated each client at discharge and reported that, compared to other clients, the HARPs were significantly more motivated in treatment, had been more punctual in attending therapy appointments, were more cooperative and self-controlled, neater in appearance, showed better recovery, and were trying harder to remain sober. Twelve-month follow-up data confirmed their impressions: The HARP clients had higher rates and longer spans of abstinence from alcohol, fewer drinking episodes, and were more likely to be employed (Leake & King, 1977).

What was this amazing personality test that predicted client behavior and outcomes over a year? Well, the researchers had a secret. The HARP clients had actually been chosen at random and not on the basis of any personality test results. The only difference between HARPs and the other clients was that the program counselors were told that the HARPs had a particularly good prognosis. The counselors' expectation that HARPs would do well turned out to influence how successful these clients actually were during and after treatment.

Even when not being influenced by tricky researchers, therapists do have expectations about clients, and those expectancies play a role in outcomes in much the same way they do for teachers and coaches. How does this happen? Positive or negative expectations about clients influence how they perceive and treat clients, and can thereby become self-fulfilling prophecies (Goldstein & Shipman, 1961; Jones, 1981; Leake & King, 1977).

In this way, your expectancies can influence clients' own hopes for change (Yahne & Miller, 1999). Although hope, like motivation, is sometimes thought of as a client attribute, it is also interpersonal, emerging in the context of relationships. Inspiring and evoking hope is an important therapeutic skill (Frank, 1968; Snyder, 1994), and as with the other skills discussed in this book, hope involves both internal experience or attitude and external expression.

The Attitude of Hope

A hopeful attitude is optimism: anticipating and expecting positive change. Optimism is a choice, a benefit of the doubt. You decide to see a glass as half full rather than half empty. As illustrated by the study described at the beginning of this chapter, optimism and pessimism both have a way of coming true.

It matters, for example, that you believe in the treatment you are providing. In a series of controlled clinical trials, Nathan Azrin and colleagues compared their community reinforcement approach

(CRA) with a "traditional" treatment for people with alcohol use disorders (Azrin, 1976; Azrin, Sisson, Meyers, & Godley, 1982; Hunt & Azrin, 1973). In three successive studies, CRA was found to be far superior to traditional treatment. However, both treatments had been delivered by the same behavior therapists, who were committed to CRA and regarded traditional treatment as ineffective. In a subsequent trial (Miller, Meyers, & Tonigan, 2001), CRA and traditional disease-model treatment were delivered by different therapists who were each trained in and committed to their approach. In this case, the advantage of CRA was modest at 6-month follow-up, with no difference in outcome by 18 and 24 months. Belief in what you're doing matters and is conveyed to your clients. This has been called the "Mecca effect" in that it harnesses the power of passionate believers (B. F. Shaw, 1999). It is not fully clear just how these beliefs are translated into treatment outcome, but therapist allegiance to a particular approach may increase clients' adherence to the treatment and their own confidence that it will be successful (McLeod, 2009).

Optimism and pessimism both have a way of coming true.

Some clients may particularly challenge an attitude of sustained optimism. In the course of treating a client, you may be disappointed, yet your hope need not diminish. It is common for people to cycle several (or many) times through the transtheoretical stages of contemplation, preparation, action, and maintenance before reaching stable change or recovery. Binary thinking about outcomes underestimates the vast range of benevolent changes that lie in between total "success" or "failure" (Miller, Walters, & Bennett, 2001). "Two steps forward and one step back" seems to be human nature. It is also worth considering that the benefit a client derives from your work together may not be apparent while you are still in the picture. People often describe previous therapists (or mentors, teachers, parents, or friends) who contributed critically to their lives without realizing it. Remember this when holding onto hope for a client.

The *How* of Promoting Hope

One of the earliest controlled trials of a psychological treatment was conducted in 1784 by Benjamin Franklin. Then living in Paris, he was asked by the king of France to investigate the practices of one Anton Mesmer, a hypnotist who claimed to heal physical and mental illnesses by manipulating "animal magnetism," an invisible fluid allegedly found throughout nature. "His patients increased rapidly," Franklin reported. "His cures were numerous and of the most astonishing nature" (Franklin, 1785, p. xii). Franklin's commission designed a clever series of experiments to test Mesmer's theory. Although Mesmer himself declined to participate, other practitioners of mesmerism were willing. Because Mesmer's disciples could allegedly magnetize people (and also animate and inanimate objects) without touching them, patients were blindfolded for the first version of what has subsequently been called a balanced placebo experiment (Rohsenow & Marlatt, 1981). The dramatic healing effects that were observed during face-to-face visual contact also occurred when blindfolded patients were led to believe that they were being magnetized, even when there was no therapist present. On the other hand, no effects at all were observed when a therapist exerted "magnetism" a foot and a half away from a blindfolded patient, as long as she or he was unaware of the mesmerist's presence. Similar results were found when individuals were exposed to several trees or basins of water, only one of which had been secretly "magnetized" by mesmerism. Dramatic results occurred, but were not specifically associated with the magnetized object. Franklin reflected that:

> this new agent might be no other than the imagination itself, whose power is as extensive as it is little known. . . . The imagination of sick persons has unquestionably a very frequent and considerable share in the cure of their diseases. . . . In [the physical world] as well as religion, [we] are saved by faith . . . under the genial influence of hope. Hope is an essential constituent of human life. (1785, pp. 100, 102)

Mesmer was subsequently dismissed as a fraud and banned from practicing in Paris. The fact remained, however, that Franklin had observed "numerous and astonishing" cures; they were just unrelated to Mesmer's hypothesized therapeutic mechanism.

What can you do to evoke clients' hope? Your own belief in the efficacy of treatment matters, and such positive expectancies are apparently contagious, as illustrated by the study of George Leake and Albert King (1977) described earlier. Sometimes when clients lack hope, you can lend them some of yours. Your hope may be communicated implicitly in a myriad of subtle ways, but you can also be explicit in fostering positive expectations.

CLIENT: This exposure stuff sounds hard. I'm not sure I want to do it.

THERAPIST: I understand. You're accustomed to avoiding things that trigger your fears, and here I am encouraging you to do just the opposite, to face them directly. Is it OK if I tell you why I think it's worth it?

CLIENT: OK.

THERAPIST: First of all, there is solid research showing that this works. It has been thoroughly studied in several different countries, and it really does help people get past what they fear. Avoiding feels perfectly natural, but it actually strengthens the fear and prolongs your suffering. Does that make sense to you?

CLIENT: I guess so. How long does treatment take?

THERAPIST: Well that's another advantage. There are other methods that might help you gradually over time, but with this approach we usually see good results within a few weeks.

CLIENT: Like no pain, no gain?

THERAPIST: You've got the right idea. Doing something difficult in the short run can help you have a better life in the long run. I wouldn't ask you to do something uncomfortable if I didn't think it would work, and I believe you can do it. And there's one more thing.

CLIENT: What's that?

THERAPIST: I'm not just relying on research I've read. I've been using this method for more than 10 years now. I was trained by one of the best therapists in this field, and I've used this approach with dozens of people over the years. I've seen first-hand how well and how quickly it can work, and I believe it could really help you.

CLIENT: What if it doesn't?

THERAPIST: As I said, this is not the only treatment available, and there are other things we could try. I do believe, though, that this is the best thing for us to try first, and if it doesn't happen to work for you, then I will stay with you until we find what does. Now, what questions do you have about this approach?

The therapist here offers several hopeful messages. One is an appraisal of the scientific evidence base for the proposed treatment, which encourages general efficacy. She describes her own experience, confidence, and results in using this treatment. She offers her belief that the client can do it, supporting self-efficacy. Finally, she does not hold out this treatment as the only possible hope, and reassures the client that together they will find what works.

Of course, clinical judgment is needed, and overzealous attempts to instill hope may clash with clients' own views, damaging therapeutic credibility and alliance (Constantino, Glass, Arnkoff, Ametrano, & Smith, 2011). As with other therapeutic skills, efforts to convey hope must be balanced against other skills such as empathy and collaboration.

Beyond sharing your own hope, some specific methods for enhancing clients' positive expectancies have been described in both cognitive-behavior therapy (Cheavens, Feldman, Woodward, & Snyder, 2006; Snyder et al., 2000) and motivational interviewing (Miller & Rollnick, 2013). One common strategy is to ask about difficult changes that a client has managed to make successfully in the past, and how she or he did it. Another approach is focusing on client strengths. For example, "Characteristics of Successful Changers" is an arbitrary list of 100 positive attributes, on which clients are asked to circle some adjectives that accurately describe them (Miller et al., 2019; Miller & Rollnick, 2013). You can then interview your clients about their strengths, such as in the example below.

THERAPIST: I see that you circled "persistent" here. In what ways are you a persistent person?

CLIENT: Once I decide to do something, I stick with it. You might say I'm stubborn.

THERAPIST: You don't give up easily. Give me a good example.

CLIENT: Well, I bought some clothing at a store a few months ago, some underwear actually, that was expensive but was supposed to last. It all stretched out to like three sizes too large. I went back to the store and they said I had to contact the manufacturer, so I did.

THERAPIST: What happened?

CLIENT: At first, I only found an online complaint form, so I filled it out and got a "Sorry—call us" reply with a phone number. So, I called them, and they gave me a claim number and told me to return it. I sent it in, kept the receipt, and waited. About 2 months went by, and I kept calling with the claim number. Finally, they asked what I would like in exchange, and after 2 more weeks the replacement came in the mail.

THERAPIST: It took quite a while, and you stuck with it. It sounds like you may be patient as well, willing to keep on trying.

CLIENT: Yeah, I was ticked off with how long it was taking, but I knew it wasn't the fault of the person I was talking to.

THERAPIST: You know how to keep your cool, and that chewing out the person on the phone wouldn't do any good.

CLIENT: I wouldn't like it if I had that job.

THERAPIST: You can also put yourself in someone else's place, and imagine how they feel.

CLIENT: Sure. I just wanted a fair exchange.

THERAPIST: And by being persistent, you got it.

As discussed in Chapter 5 on affirmation, strengths are something more than specific actions. You are pointing to enduring qualities of the *person,* strengths that he or she could use in many different situations.

Biases That Can Work against Therapist Optimism

As we noted previously, it is important in facilitating clients' hope to retain optimism in your own expectations about client outcomes (Martin, Sterne, Moore, & Friedmeyer, 1976; Martin, Moore, & Sterne, 1977). Therapists face a professional hazard here because of the sampling bias in people presenting for treatment. In therapeutic practice, one typically sees mostly clients who have been unable to make needed changes, rather than the many who have successfully changed with or without the help of therapists (Snyder, Michael, & Cheavens, 1999). When you're daily confronted with clients who have failed at such efforts, you can lose confidence in the potential for people to change. One privilege of doing treatment outcome research is following up with everyone who has been treated. In doing clinical trials, we have been impressed with how well most people fare after treatment of substance use disorders. We have remained in addiction treatment for decades because the outcomes are so encouraging, but one might not appreciate this if only working in an intake service (Miller, Forcehimes, & Zweben, 2019).

Another potential negative information bias is that by training, behavioral health professionals tend to look for pathology, while overlooking clients' strengths and positive qualities (Stack, Lannon, & Miley, 1983). There is vibrant and reassuring scholarship on the remarkable resilience of human beings even after trauma, torture, misfortune, and childhood deprivation (Rutter, 2006, 2013). If your daily work immerses you in pathology and heartbreak, knowledge of human resilience and of overall positive treatment outcomes can be spirit-saving, and reinforce your sense of optimism.

Research on Hope

The potency of a placebo effect is well documented (A. K. Shapiro, 1971; Wampold, Minami, Tierney, Baskin, & Bhati, 2005). Though sometimes maligned, as if a trick were being played on clients, placebos illustrate the benevolent effect of hope in healing. On a smaller scale, self-efficacy (belief in one's ability to succeed in a particular task) similarly presages success (Bandura, 1997) and can be enhanced by behavioral interventions (French, Olander, Chisholm, & McSharry, 2014; O'Halloran, Shields, Blackstock, Wintle, & Taylor, 2016; Prestwich et al., 2014; Sheeran et al., 2016). A variety of therapist characteristics have also been linked to the evocation of client hope, including warmth, supportiveness, credibility, empathy, and positive regard (Howe, Goyer, & Crum, 2017; Kaptchuk et al., 2008; Orlinsky & Howard, 1986; Turner, Deyo, Loeser, Con Korff, & Fordyce, 1994).

Therapist communications can *dampen* client expectancies as well. For decades, we used waiting list groups as an ethically

esponsible control condition in clinical trials, in that all participants
ould eventually receive the treatment being studied (Miller et al.,
993; Miller & DiPilato, 1983; Schmidt & Miller, 1983). The consis-
nt finding was that clients on a waiting list showed no improvement
all until treatment was received, and then responded positively. A
rther trial (Harris & Miller, 1990) randomized clients with alco-
ol use disorder to immediate outpatient treatment, or a single ses-
on providing encouragement and a self-help manual, or a waiting
t control condition. The finding was familiar: Both intervention
oups had substantial reductions in drinking by 10 weeks, whereas
ose on the waiting list showed no change in drinking until they
ceived outpatient treatment (see Figure 8.1).

Why would those on a waiting list show no change even though
ey had presented themselves for treatment, had completed pre-
atment assessment, and self-identified their drinking problems?
simple explanation is that they did what they were told to do.
ey waited. When telling clients that they are on a waiting list,
e implicit instruction is that they are not expected to get better,
at there is nothing they can or need to do until they receive treat-
nt. In contrast, those in the brief intervention self-change condi-
n were told to get started right away on changing their drinking,

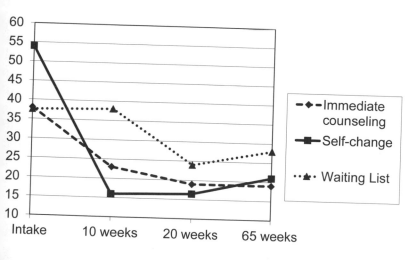

RE 8.1. Random assignment to immediate treatment, self-change, or
ing list.

using guidelines provided in a self-help book (the same content as wa
being offered in outpatient counseling), and check back with us in 1
weeks. In this sense, telling clients they are on a waiting list can b
pernicious, undermining even natural change efforts (Miller, 2015

Waiting for behavior change is no

---

*Telling clients they are on a
waiting list can be pernicious.*

---

like waiting for needed surgery.
is better to offer something rig
away that is likely to be helpf
and that empowers personal agency (Cheavens et al., 2006). Even
placebo intervention can yield more positive change than a waitir
list (Kaptchuk et al., 2008).

The power of therapist expectancies is enough of an influen
that researchers make efforts to measure and account for it in clinic
trials. As discussed earlier, when therapists are allied with a trea
ment, it is more likely to be successful, as opposed to when they a
offering treatment they do not believe in (Falkenström, Markowi
Jonker, Philips, & Holmqvist, 2013). Beyond this allegiance effe
other research has shown that therapists' expectations of clier
prognosis are good predictors of their actual outcomes (Katz
Hoyt, 2014; P. J. Martin et al., 1977; Norris et al., 2019). Are the
pists simply good "prophets," or do their beliefs actually influer
outcomes? To our knowledge, this is a question that has not be
addressed with experimental studies in psychosocial interventio
other than the clever study by Leake and King (1977) described
the beginning of this chapter. The answer to this question may dir
depending on the client and the presenting problem (Strauss, H
pert, Simpson, & Foa, 2018), and therapist expectancies may ma
less in some situations than in others. Still, based on the robust
erature concerning the powerful effects of teacher's expectations
students (Rosenthal & Jacobson, 1966; Rubies-Davis & Rosent
2016; Szumski & Karwowski, 2019), we think it is reasonable
suppose that initial expectations have a role in influencing outcon
rather than simply being a reflection of the therapist's astutenes
prediction. In a study with 167 psychodynamic therapists, pessim
was associated with the most negative client outcomes (Sandell et
2006). This makes therapeutic optimism worth careful cultivat
Indeed, it would be unusual if optimism in a therapist were diffe
from other human relationships, where it is a cherished commo
in mentors, coaches, parents, friends, and partners.

KEY POINTS

- Clients' hope and expectancy (sometimes called a placebo effect) are associated with better health and treatment outcomes.
- Therapists' beliefs about client prognosis can become self-fulfilling prophecies.
- Therapist beliefs about the treatment procedures being used also influence outcomes.
- Specific clinical procedures can increase or decrease clients' expectations for change.
- Placement on a "waiting list" appears to be an efficacious instruction not to change.

CHAPTER 9

Evocation

Not only therapists but also clients bring important strengths and expertise to the change process (Bohart & Tallman, 1999; Wampold & Imel, 2015). In fact, client attributes are at least as important as therapist characteristics and skills in accounting for overall psychotherapy outcomes (Duncan, Miller, Wampold, & Hubble, 2010). Clients with more motivation for change, engagement, hope, and self-efficacy tend to have better prognoses. Yet, these are not static traits; they emerge in the interpersonal context of treatment, and their expression can be influenced by what you do.

In this chapter, we address evocation as a skill not often included in lists of therapeutic factors that influence client outcomes. Evocation calls forth and supports what clients already have, their own strengths and wisdom. Your client becomes a collaborator in the process of change. Evocation can be thought of as facilitating clients' own self-healing potential (Bohart & Tallman, 1999, 2010; Levitt & Pomerville, 2016).

The ability to evoke a client's own resources is a particular skill of therapists that stands in contrast to the technical skills of teaching and advising. It is not necessary to choose between evocation and direction; a guiding style encompasses both (Miller & Rollnick, 2013), and emerging research on responsiveness indicates that the balance of evoking and advising is best adjusted according to client characteristics (C. J. Edwards, Beutler, & Someah, 2019; Karno

& Longabaugh, 2005). Effective therapists can balance directional strategies with calling forth the client's own assets for change. As with the other interpersonal skills discussed in this book, evocation encompasses both the clinician's internal attitude and corresponding external behaviors.

The Attitude of Evocation

A starting point in the attitude of evocation is recognizing that there *is* something important to evoke from clients. An opposite pole from that attitude is perceiving oneself as the expert who provides what clients do not have or cannot do themselves. Some forms of psychotherapy heavily emphasize giving clients something that they lack, be it insight, knowledge, skills, motivation, or rational thinking. Evocation assumes strengths rather than deficits. Instead of saying implicitly, "I have what you need and I'm going to give it to you," the message in evocation is, "You have what you need, and together we're going to find it."

Yes, you have hard-won expertise from your professional training and experience, and offering that expertise is part of a helping relationship (Chapter 10). Clients also have vital expertise. As discussed at the end of Chapter 1, no one knows more about your clients than they do. Figuring out how to incorporate change into an ongoing life is a collaborative, not a prescriptive, process. It is your clients who ultimately decide whether, why, when, and how to change. Part of the underlying attitude of evocation, then, is viewing counseling and psychotherapy as a collaborative partnership, not an expert operation with the client as a passive recipient. Clients become active participants in change.

> *Evocation: "You have what you need, and together we're going to find it."*

Curiosity is also part of an evoking attitude. You not only assume that your clients have important resourcefulness and gifts; you are eager to discover them. You don't know in advance what any particular client will bring to the helping relationship. There can be a sense of wonder in this, a prizing of your clients' wisdom and strengths.

Your own contribution to evocation further involves knowing what to evoke. What is important for clients to verbalize and experience during counseling? This is guided, in part, by your implicit model of human nature and change, and also by available research on therapeutic process. We will describe two evidence-based forms of evocation in therapy, but we turn first to some practical tools for evoking.

The *How* of Evocation

What your clients say during treatment does not occur in a vacuum, but in interacting with you. In some forms of counseling and psychotherapy, helpers encourage particular kinds of speech (e.g., free associations, catharsis, expression of feelings, positive expectancies) that are presumed to lead to healing or growth. Depending on one's theoretical model, these optimal forms of speech might be invited by asking questions, empathic reflection, flooding, or unrelenting silence. Therapeutic methods may be consciously strategic (Haley, 1993; R. J. Kohlenberg & Tsai, 2007), or conceptualized simply as therapeutic conditions for natural healing to occur (Rogers, 1959; Truax & Carkhuff, 1967).

You may or may not be conscious of why you ask particular questions, reflect or affirm specific content, or form summaries as you do. Whether or not therapists are aware of the process, some form of evocation occurs in virtually all types of counseling and psychotherapy. Differences arise in what therapists seek to evoke, and how they go about it. One counselor we coached, for example, initially practiced as if it is therapeutic for clients to describe in great detail their most negative emotions, and the adverse experiences in their past and current lives. Focusing instead on clients' values, goals, and strengths dramatically improved his clients' experience during sessions, and their willingness to continue in counseling.

Perhaps the simplest understanding of evocation is embedded in the idea that, in counseling, you are likely to hear more of whatever you focus on and pay attention to. Specific counseling "microskills" can be used to invite and emphasize certain aspects of what clients say. Four such microskills that have been applied and studied in motivational interviewing are represented by the mnemonic acronym OARS: Open question, Affirmation, Reflection, and Summary (Miller & Rollnick, 2013).

Questions anticipate and require an answer, and in that sense are directive. Closed questions ask for a specific piece of information like a number, date, or address. Open questions give clients greater latitude to respond:

- "What brings you here today and how do you hope we might help?"
- "What do you enjoy most about your relationship?"
- "If our work together were 100% successful, what would be different?"
- "Tell me about your mother."

When you ask a question, you direct the client's (and your) attention. What you ask indicates what you regard to be important. It matters what you ask.

Affirmation (Chapter 5) means commenting positively on some aspect of a client's statements, actions, or attributes. For better or worse, you are likely to hear more of whatever you affirm (Karpiak & Benjamin, 2004). It matters what clients say in treatment, and it matters what you affirm.

Reflections (Chapter 3) focus attention on particular aspects of what a client has said. They can function as a form of positive reinforcement (Truax, 1966). You are likely to hear more about whatever you reflect, and clients' own attention is thereby directed to consider the content further. It matters what you reflect.

Summaries pull together what a client has said and what has transpired. Yet, summaries seldom include everything that has been said and done; they focus attention on specific aspects that are important enough to include. It matters what you put into a summary.

All four of these microskills influence what clients will and won't say during counseling, which, in turn, presages treatment outcome. Sequential analyses of counseling sessions reveal the extent to which particular therapist responses elicit or reinforce client responses (Bischoff & Tracey, 1995; Drage, Masterson, Tober, Farragher, & Bewick, 2019; Klonek, Lehmann-Willenbrock, & Kauffeld, 2014; Moyers et al., 2007; Walthers et al., 2019; Wiser & Goldfried, 1998).

> *Microskills influence what clients say, which, in turn, presages treatment outcome.*

A common measure of evocation (though not the only one) is language that the client uses during a clinical interaction. Positive outcomes after treatment are predictable from the extent to which clients verbalize more of certain things during sessions (such as motivation, self-exploration, self-efficacy, or commitment) and less of others (such as argumentativeness or hopelessness). The kinds of client speech that are regarded to be optimal vary across systems of psychotherapy, but the general assertion here is that what clients say during treatment is *malleable* and contains important information about their likely outcome. Ideally, the client speech to be evoked is:

1. observable and reliably measurable
2. variable enough to be useful—neither always nor rarely present
3. responsive to therapeutic communications, and
4. empirically linked to treatment outcome.

These characteristics of in-session language can be studied in psycholinguistic research linking therapist and client speech with subsequent outcomes. We offer two examples of client speech that meet these criteria: "experiencing" and "change talk." They are observable, variable, responsive to therapist skill, and predict better treatment outcome.

Two Examples of Therapeutic Evocation

Experiencing

Traditionally prized within a person-centered approach are client expressions of feelings and here-and-now experiences, more than superficial generalities, impersonal observations, or intellectual abstraction. The construct of *experiencing* emerged within person-centered counseling, focusing on the depth of clients' emotional engagement in therapy (Gendlin, 1961; Rogers et al., 1967) and their ability to bring their own searching and concern into the interaction with the therapist (Bugental, 1999). Client experiencing (EXP) has typically been measured on a 7-point ordinal rating scale, with specific descriptions of each of seven "stages" of phenomenological self-exploration (M. H. Klein, Mathieu-Coughlan, & Kiesler, 1986).

EXP ratings are based solely on the client's own verbalizations and particularly reflect spoken self-disclosure (Stiles, McDaniel, & Gaughey, 1979). At the low end, clients' experiencing is superficial, impersonal, and devoid of personal emotion. First-person pronouns are rare. At midpoint, clients are more introspective. Rather than giving detached descriptive accounts of events, they recount feelings and a personal perspective. In other words, they convey their own experience of events. Higher ratings reflect ongoing awareness and exploration of immediate and emergent experiences. These in-session ratings are meant to reflect clients' potential introspective depth of experiencing. Reported interrater reliabilities of EXP after coder training have been high (M. H. Klein et al., 1986; Watson & Bedard, 2006).

A relatively consistent finding is that in-session depth of client EXP predicts better treatment outcome (Hill, 1990; Luborsky, Auerbach, Chandler, Cohen, & Bachrach, 1971; Orlinsky & Howard, 1986; Pascuel-Leone & Yervomenko, 2017; Watson & Bedard, 2006; Wiser & Goldfried, 1998). This predictive relationship has been observed within various therapeutic contexts including marital (Johnson & Greenberg, 1988) and brief psychotherapy (Hill et al., 1988), cognitive (Castonguay, Goldfried, Wiser, Raue, & Hayes, 1996), experiential (Goldman, Greenberg, & Pos, 2005; Watson & Bedard, 2006) and emotion-focused therapy (Robichaud, 2004), and in clients with and without schizophrenia (Kiesler, 1971; Rogers et al., 1967).

How, then, can therapists facilitate clients' experiencing? In a Wisconsin trial (Rogers et al., 1967), two of the three therapeutic conditions (empathy and genuineness) did predict deeper client in-session EXP, which, in turn, predicted more favorable outcomes. Subsequent studies have yielded more mixed results when examining aggregate levels of therapist conditions (M. H. Klein et al., 1986). Accurate empathy (Chapter 3) would seem a good candidate, in that reflections often focus on the client's experiences, feelings, and meaning (Elliott et al., 2011a). Even here, though, observed relationships have been relatively weak and inconsistent between therapists' level of in-session empathy and client EXP.

Because counselor and client behavior are interdependent (Hill, 2005), sequential analyses of in-session responses may offer a finer-grained picture of their relationship. This happens when researchers pay attention to the order of what clients and therapists say to each other, rather than looking at the overall correlation of their speech. In sequential research, what a client says immediately after a therapist speaks (and the reverse) is examined, and conditional probabilities are generated. From these, one can calculate the probability that a particular kind of speech (such as EXP) will occur when a therapist offers, for example, a reflection of feeling. This can help form hypotheses about what might cause clients to "upshift" or "downshift" in EXP during therapy sessions.

Susan Wiser and Marvin Goldfried (1998) used utterance-by-utterance coding to study therapist responses that predicted client experiencing in psychodynamic and cognitive-behavior therapy. Interestingly, no therapist behavior or orientation was systematically associated with clients shifting from low EXP (1–3 on the 7-point scale) to higher EXP levels (4 or above). However, therapist responses did differentiate whether clients would sustain high EXP or shift down to low EXP in sessions. More affirming, accepting, and empathic therapist responses favored clients' continuing in high EXP. Downshifting to low EXP occurred when therapists talked more and (particularly in cognitive-behavior therapy) with a more interpersonally controlling therapeutic style.

Clients' average EXP ratings may also vary across therapeutic orientations that place different amounts of emphasis on emotional experiencing. Comparative studies have reported higher EXP levels in experiential rather than either cognitive-behavioral (Watson & Bedard, 2006) or client-centered therapy (Watson & Greenberg, 1996), and no EXP differences between cognitive-behavioral and psychodynamic psychotherapy (Wiser & Goldfried, 1998). Average experiencing ratings can be significantly increased by directly instructing clients in the characteristics of high EXP responses (M. H. Klein et al., 1986), for example, by encouraging clients to attend to their emotions explicitly, or to linger when they are bypassing emotionally meaningful events.

Emotional experiencing, then, is a reliably measurable client factor predictive of outcome across a variety of therapeutic approaches. EXP is theoretically important in client-centered and other experiential therapies, and is differentially responsive to therapeutic practices. Sequential process research with EXP is at an early stage, and is needed to determine what therapist responses are more likely to foster or hinder it regardless of theoretical orientation. Based on research to date, the therapist skills described in Chapters 3–6 (empathy, acceptance, positive regard, and genuineness) encourage clients to sustain higher levels of EXP during treatment.

Change Talk

At first glance, the idea that a client's language during treatment sessions would predict change may seem odd. After all, people often say things they don't mean, or promise to do things they don't intend to do. Yet, there is good reason to suppose that what clients say in a treatment session can actually shape their beliefs and subsequent behaviors. Mood induction research (M. Martin, 1990; Westermann, Spies, Stahl, & Hesse, 1996) illustrates how spoken words can elicit emotional states. Stating an intention to take a specific action increases the likelihood of doing it (Gollwitzer, 1999; Gollwitzer, Wieber, Myers, & McCrea, 2010). Self-described values can shape subsequent action (Rokeach, 1973; Sherman, 2013). Counter-attitudinal role-play—publicly defending a perspective that is opposite to one's own—results in an attitude shift toward the defended position, provided it was uncoerced (Bem, 1967; Festinger, 1957). Spoken words matter.

This in itself is probably not surprising to you. What is often underestimated, however, is the extent to which you shape your clients' speech. Consciously or not, you do influence the content of your clients' in-session speech by the particular questions you ask, what you choose to affirm or to highlight with reflective listening, and what you put into summaries (DeVargas & Stormshak, 2020; Glynn & Moyers, 2010; Miller & Rollnick, 2013). It matters what you encourage clients to say.

This complex interaction of clinician and client speech may account, in part, for the large differences among therapists' outcomes, over and above the impact of general therapeutic factors such as empathy. For example, persistently asking about and reflecting negative affect would be expected to worsen a client's depressed mood. A distressed couple is unlikely to be helped by allowing them in session to continue voicing their grievances and defending their resentments toward each other.

Selective use of questions and reflections can be conscious and strategic. Solution-focused therapy, for example, invokes a future-oriented, problem-solving focus rather than dwelling on the past (Berg & Reuss, 1997; deShazer et al., 2007). In functional analytic psychotherapy, the therapist consciously reinforces in-session clinically relevant behaviors linked to positive change (B. S. Kohlenberg, Yeater, & Kohlenberg, 1998; R. J. Kohlenberg & Tsai, 1994). In such approaches, the therapist is consciously attending to and evoking client speech to move toward a particular outcome.

Within an explicitly client-centered approach, motivational interviewing pays particular attention to clients' statements that express personal motivation for and commitment to change. The idea of such self-motivational statements was originally linked to Daryl Bem's (1967, 1972) self-perception theory: that you learn what you believe as you hear yourself speak (Miller, 1983). In essence, people literally talk themselves into or out of change by verbalizing their own pro-change and counter-change motivations (Miller & Rollnick, 2004). Speech acts favoring change ("change talk"; Amrhein, Miller, Yahne, Knupsky, & Hochstein, 2004; Miller & Rollnick, 2013) can take many forms, including:

> desire (I want, wish, would like)
> ability (I can, could, am able)
> reasons (if . . . then)
> need (I have to, must, need to), and
> commitment (I will, promise, have decided)

Counter-change verbalizations ("sustain talk") represent the opposite pole of ambivalence and can take the same forms of speech (I don't want, can't, don't need to, etc.).

This would be of modest interest except for the fact that treatment outcomes are associated with such specific types of speech. Client change talk predicts subsequent positive behavior change outcomes, particularly when measured in proportion to sustain talk—that is, client arguments against change (Amrhein, Miller, Yahne, Palmer, & Fulcher, 2003; Bertholet, Faouzi, Gmel, Gaume, & Daeppen, 2010; S. D. Campbell et al., 2010; Daeppen, Bertholet, Gmel, & Gaume, 2007; M. Magill, Apodaca, Barnett, & Monti, 2010; Moyers, Martin, et al., 2007; Moyers, Houck, et al., 2017; Vader et al., 2010). In the clinical method of motivational interviewing, counselors particularly attend to, seek to evoke, and consciously reflect change talk in order to strengthen it (Apodaca et al., 2016; Drage et al., 2019; Gaume, Bertholet, Faouzi, Gmel, & Daeppen, 2010; Glynn & Moyers, 2010; Miller & Rollnick, 2013; Miller & Rose, 2009; Moyers, Houck, et al., 2017). In a social work study of child protective interventions, family outcomes were directly predicted by workers' evocation skills (Forrester et al, 2019).

What does it look like when clinicians are actively trying to evoke client language about change? Here is an example:

THERAPIST: You mentioned that your doctor told you to get more exercise, and I'm interested in your own thoughts and feelings about this. What do you think might be some advantages of increasing your physical activity? *An open question, the usual answer to which would be change talk.*

CLIENT: I would probably feel better. *Change talk*

THERAPIST: In what ways do you think you might feel better? *Asking for elaboration of change talk that the client has offered*

CLIENT: Stronger maybe? I know if I just let my body go, it's downhill from there. *Change talk*

THERAPIST: Like use it or lose it. *Reflection*

CLIENT: Right. I'd rather not be disabled as I get older. *Change talk*

THERAPIST: Being more active could keep you stronger, more able to do things you enjoy. How else might you feel better? *Reflection* / *Open question*

CLIENT: I would probably have more energy. After work and dinner, I feel exhausted and just watch TV. *Change talk*

THERAPIST: Kind of a vicious cycle there; you feel run down and so don't do much other than watch TV in the evening. *Reflection*

CLIENT: Even on the weekend.

THERAPIST: So, being more active could help you stay stronger, not get disabled over time, and have more energy to do what you enjoy. What might be some other good things about getting more exercise? *Summary of change talk so far*

Open question

CLIENT: Maybe I would sleep better. But I don't like the idea of exercise. It's so boring. *Change talk, then sustain talk*

THERAPIST: Whatever you would do to be more active, you don't want it to be boring or to think of it as "exercise." What kinds of activity have you enjoyed? *Reflection (of sustain talk)*

Open question shifts back the focus to change

CLIENT: I used to like tennis. I just kind of let tennis go when I started feeling so tired.

THERAPIST: I see—tennis is something that you might enjoy again. *Reflection*

CLIENT: Yes, I guess I could. *Change talk*

THERAPIST: So, never mind the word "exercise." What else might be good about being more physically active in your everyday life? *Open question*

CLIENT: The doctor said I could stand to lose some weight. *Change talk*

THERAPIST: What might that do for you? *Open question*

CLIENT: My blood pressure has been getting high, and I don't want to take medication.   *Change talk*

THERAPIST: You like being self-reliant. You want to do it on your own, to know that it's your own effort that's making the difference.   *Affirmation* / *Reflection*

CLIENT: Right. I think I can get my blood pressure down without taking meds.   *Change talk*

THERAPIST: And tennis or other physical activity could help you do that.   *Reflection (continuing the paragraph)*

CLIENT: Yes, I think so, and cutting down salt.   *Change talk*

THERAPIST: So, you're somebody who really wants to stay healthy, and you know some things you can do to make that happen.   *Affirmation*

What would you be willing to try, to be more active in your daily life?   *Open question*

CLIENT: I could go back to the playing tennis on the weekend. I think I'd like that.   *Change talk*

THERAPIST: Sounds good! That's something you could do on weekends.   *Affirmation*

What might you try on weekdays instead of TV?   *Open question*

CLIENT: You know, I used to walk up in the foothills. It's not far from my house. I could do that in the morning before I go to work. I know that's not replacing TV at night, but I would enjoy it.   *Change talk*

THERAPIST: That's something you could try without much preparation. It's nice up there most days. So, tennis, walking in the morning before work; these could help you stay strong, have more energy, maybe lose a bit of weight, and be able to do what you enjoy.   *Summary of change talk*

CLIENT: And maybe at night I could take a walk after dinner. . . .   *Change talk*

If the therapist had started prescribing exercise, this conversation could have turned out quite differently. Instead, he got curious and asked open questions, the expected answer to which would be change talk. He reflected what the client said, offered some affirmation, and gave short summaries of the client's own change talk.

In this form of evocation, you invite clients to describe their motivations for and ideas about change, reflect and affirm what they say, and pull it together. In that way, your clients hear themselves voice their own change talk; then they hear it again when you reflect it, and again if you weave it into a summary. You are quite literally helping people talk themselves into change (Miller & Rollnick, 2004).

Counselor Restraint

Much of this book is about what effective therapists do, but it is also worth considering what to refrain from doing, or at least to practice in moderation. Informal "chat" that is off-topic can undermine therapeutic progress and motivation for change (Bamatter et al., 2010). Criticizing (telling people what is wrong with them), advising, and directing (telling people what to do) tend to evoke defensiveness, which, in turn, predicts non-adherence and a lack of subsequent change (Apodaca et al., 2016; de Almeida Neto, 2017; M. Magill, Bernstein, et al., 2019; Patterson & Forgatch, 1985). This is particularly true when clients are verbally defensive, hostile, or oppositional (Karno & Longabaugh, 2005).

Counseling in a way that evokes client resistance and defense of the status quo can hinder positive change. This may happen with the best of intentions when you try to urge clients in the right direction. When someone is ambivalent about change and you champion the pro-change arguments, a normal response is to voice the other side, the counter-change arguments. Let's see how the conversation above might have gone very differently if the therapist had advocated for exercise instead of evoking the client's own arguments for change.

> THERAPIST: You really do need to get more exercise. [directing]
>
> CLIENT: I just don't like exercising.
>
> THERAPIST: But it's important to your long-term health. If you don't stay active, you will lose your muscle mass over time. [warning]
>
> CLIENT: Exercise is boring, and besides, I'm tired after work.
>
> THERAPIST: Maybe you could do something in the morning before work. [advising]
>
> CLIENT: Look, I work hard. I'm already up at 6:30 and I don't want to get less sleep.

See what's happening here? By making the pro-change arguments, the therapist is evoking defensive sustain talk. Both arguments were already there inside the client. Which arguments the client will voice depends on how you conduct the conversation, and people are most likely to be persuaded by what they hear themselves say.

Counseling in a way that evokes client defense of the status quo can hinder positive change.

Similarly, the communication roadblocks to good listening (described in Chapter 3) tend to derail clients from exploring their own experience. Roadblocks are often done with good intentions, even when trying to listen, but they do divert clients from experiencing.

> CLIENT: I just feel so nervous about this upcoming meeting.
>
> THERAPIST: I'm sure you'll do fine. [reassuring]
>
> CLIENT: Well, I'm not so sure.
>
> THERAPIST: It's worse when you're anticipating the event, imagining what it will be like, than it is when it's actually happening. [analyzing]

CLIENT: You don't know how hard this is for me!

THERAPIST: Actually, I do. [persuading]

CLIENT: How could you know what it's like for me?

THERAPIST: I used to be very nervous about public speaking. Just focus on what you know, and it will go well. [advising]

This might be sound advice, but the conversation is no longer about what the client is experiencing. Effective therapists exercise restraint with such roadblocks.

How might this conversation be different if the therapist avoided roadblocks and prioritized evoking instead?

CLIENT: I just feel so nervous about this upcoming meeting.

THERAPIST: It's your old fear that you told me about; that you won't be able to speak and others will think you are stupid. [empathic reflection]

CLIENT: Even though I've practiced the relaxation and visualization you taught me, I'm still kind of stressing.

THERAPIST: You're better prepared than in the past because of the work you've been doing. [recognizing change talk and reflecting it]

CLIENT: I've spent hours and hours doing those exercises, so that *should* help. I guess I will find out—but what if it doesn't?

THERAPIST: You are like an athlete at the starting block, wondering how the race will go. [reframing anxiety]

CLIENT: Actually, that's a good point. Maybe everyone feels nervous before the big competition. I guess I'm not that different.

Other Forms of Evocation

Evoking could be focused on any kind of speech that clients offer during sessions that is deemed to facilitate positive change. For example, self-efficacy is a widely studied correlate of behavior change (Bandura, 1982, 1997) that can be increased by various experimental, training, and clinical interventions (French et al., 2014; Gist & Mitchell, 1992;

Williams & French, 2011). Furthermore, interventions that increase self-efficacy can, in turn, impact behavioral intentions and change (Prestwich et al., 2014; Sheeran et al., 2016). To date, little research has focused on strategically evoking clients' in-session self-efficacy speech. The psycholinguistic studies of motivational interviewing described above have included *ability* verbalizations as one form of change talk, and Miller and Rollnick (2013) have proposed specific procedures to elicit client confidence regarding change. Causal links between particular therapist responses and client self-efficacy speech remain to be demonstrated.

Research on Evoking

Demonstration of the therapeutic value of evocation involves two components. First, it should be demonstrated that the speech of interest is relevant, by predicting subsequent positive change or treatment outcome. Here, the evidence for client language is strong (Houck, Manuel, & Moyers, 2018; M. Magill et al., 2018). A predominance of client sustain talk predicts worse outcomes, whereas a higher proportion of change talk predicts better outcomes. This is not very interesting in itself, for it might simply mean that clients who speak against change are unmotivated and so don't end up changing, whereas those who are more motivated speak more positively about change and carry through. In other words, we might be measuring the smoke (client language) instead of the fire (motivation) that produced it.

What is more telling is the second step, which shows that therapist responses are closely associated with clients' language. When therapists are affirming, use reflection, and avoid direction and coercion, clients offer more change talk (and experiencing), and less sustain talk (DeVargas & Stormshak, 2020). If language were simply a passive marker of something that the client carries into the room (a moderating variable), there should not be this kind of correlation between therapist action and changes in language. Of course, correlations like these in themselves do not establish causality, in that client responses may also elicit counselor responses, or some third factor may account for their interrelationship. As noted earlier, sequential coding is more promising, yielding conditional probabilities of particular client verbalizations following specific counselor responses

(Hannover, Blaut, Kniehase, Martin, & Hannich, 2013; Moyers & Martin, 2006; Walthers et al., 2019). Other evidence for change talk has emerged from experimental studies in which the pertinent client responses systematically vary with randomly assigned counselor style changes (Miller et al., 1993), or in an A-B-A-B within-client design (Glynn & Moyers, 2010; Patterson & Forgatch, 1985).

Taken together, these studies argue strongly that therapists have a direct role in evoking (or suppressing) client speech about change, and that this speech is likely to have an impact on a client's treatment outcome. More generally, the ability of clinicians to draw out the client's unique resources in favor of change (including their own language) is a powerful and often neglected aspect of therapeutic expertise.

KEY POINTS

- What clients say during treatment is consequential, predicting eventual outcomes.

- You influence what clients verbalize through the questions you ask, the content you reflect and affirm, and what you include in summaries.

- Client factors such as motivation for change, engagement, hope, and self-efficacy do predict outcomes, and are likewise influenced by therapist responses.

- Evocation calls forth the client's own wisdom, strengths, and resources.

- Experiencing and change talk are two types of client speech that can be evoked by therapist responses, and are associated with better treatment outcome.

- Positive outcomes are also facilitated by what you refrain from evoking, such as "resistance" and "chat" unrelated to treatment goals.

CHAPTER 10

Offering Information and Advice

What is the role of a professional helper? Consider a spectrum of possible therapist–client relationships ranging from "directing" to "following." At one extreme is a directing style that involves telling people what they should do by dispensing information, solutions, instructions, or advice. There are times when this is an appropriate and even expected role. At the opposite extreme is a compassionate companion who listens empathically, conveys acceptance and affirmation, and assiduously avoids providing answers or advice. Sometimes this is what clients prefer. At least in stereotype, some professions lean toward the former: probation officer, diabetes educator, lawyer, sports coach, or financial advisor. The latter, again in stereotype, might be a client-centered counselor, hospice worker, or supportive friend.

In practice, most professional roles involve some combination of directing and following, of technical and relational skills. Informing and advising can easily be overdone, and may even undermine a client's own motivation (Brehm & Brehm, 1981; de Almeida Neto, 2017). Yet, physicians, attorneys, or financial advisors who merely listen without offering any advice would be shirking their duty. In between the two extremes is the role of a guide, who both listens well and provides expertise. If you travel to another country, you do not expect a guide to order you what to do, or decide what you would prefer or enjoy. Neither does a good guide merely follow you around. Even in traditionally directive professions, a guiding style can be far more effective than just telling people what to do (Rollnick, Fader, Breckon, & Moyers, 2019; Rollnick, Kaplan, & Rutschman, 2016; Rollnick et al., in 2020; Steinberg & Miller, 2015; Stinson & Clark, 2017).

A helper's first instinct is often to offer clients advice or useful information. After all, by virtue of a hard-won professional education, you have built up a storehouse of knowledge. For example, you may have well-informed hunches about why a particular client:

> Feels fatigued yet agitated, and has been losing weight
> Awakens some mornings seeing strange people in the room, and is unable to move or speak
> Gets up five times during the night to urinate
> Repeatedly falls for the same kind of romantic partner, with disastrous results
> Often misses or is late to work or school on Mondays

And having developed a provisional hypothesis regarding a client's distress, you may race ahead to think of potential solutions. Indeed, people often go to helping professionals in hopes of better understanding what they are experiencing and what to do about it.

In a classic nondirective approach, counselors would refrain from giving answers or advice. This is the structure of simplistic Carl Rogers jokes, but Rogers himself shed the concept of being nondirective for a more positive focus on being person-centered (Kirschenbaum, 2009). You may well feel a professional-ethical obligation to provide information and recommendations, and sometimes advice alone can be enough to trigger change (Aveyard, Begh, Parsons, & West, 2012; Chick, Ritson, Connaughton, & Stewart, 1988; G. Edwards et al., 1977; Schmidt & Miller, 1983).

Where is the balance? Advising is a part of your job, but the question is when and how best to do it. In professional services, information and advice are offered within the context of a helping relationship, and in that sense all of the preceding chapters apply. There is a particular pitfall to be aware of before proceeding directly to educate and advise.

Psychological Reactance

Efforts to persuade someone to change often fail and can even back-fire, producing the opposite effect from what was intended (Dillard & Shen, 2005). As described in Chapter 4, "psychological reactance" is a commonly observed resistance to persuasion and advice (J. W. Brehm, 1966; S. S. Brehm & Brehm, 1981), a "well-established inher-ent tendency to act contrary to recommendations from others . . . even where they agree" (de Almeida Neto, 2017). When personal freedom is constrained, the proscribed behavior becomes all the more attractive and more likely to occur. (Think of telling teenagers to "just say no" to drugs.) In Jack and Sharon Brehms' formulation, there is an inherent motivation to restore one's sense of autonomy and freedom of choice whenever it is threatened. This reactance may be rooted in the millennia-long evolution of social power hierarchies: to comply with advice or direction is to accept a one-down position (de Almeida Neto, 2017). Self-determination theory similarly emphasizes the importance of autonomy (as well as competence and relatedness) in human motivation (Deci & Ryan, 2008; Ryan & Deci, 2017).

Triggering the natural response of reactance is a pitfall to avoid when offering information and advice. Whatever its genesis, the social phenomenon of resistance to advice is well documented (Steindl et al., 2015), and has both cognitive and affective components (Rains, 2013). Beyond the general phe-nomenon, there are individual dif-ferences in proneness to reactance that can affect clients' sensitivity and response to therapist directive-ness (Beutler et al., 2011; Dillard & Shen, 2005; Karno & Long-abaugh, 2005).

Reactance is an "inherent tendency to act contrary to recommendations."

The Attitude of Informing and Advising

Freedom to choose is not something that you can grant to your clients. They already have it. Ultimately, it is up to them whether they will lis-ten to or ignore you, believe or disagree with information that you pro-vide, and follow or shun the advice you offer. You cannot *make* people change. They get to decide; it's a given in any helping relationship.

Knowing, accepting, and honoring clients' autonomy is an important context for whatever information and advice you provide.

A related therapeutic attitude behind information and advice is appropriate humility. Framed degrees on the wall may afford some credibility, but modesty is in order in any helping relationship about behavior and lifestyle. Communications that put you in a "one up" position often foster defensiveness and may undermine your efforts to help. Assertions that "You can't," "You must," or "You have to" are simply untrue. The usual meaning of these types of statements is a warning about adverse or dire consequences, but it is better to acknowledge a client's autonomy and consider possible choices in light of potential outcomes. We long ago found that if we told clients, "You can't drink," they would quickly prove us wrong.

> Knowing, accepting, and honoring clients' autonomy are key.

Related to humility is remembering that clients have knowledge, strengths, wisdom, and ideas of their own (Chapter 9). A helping relationship brings together your professional expertise with a client's lived experience and know-how. Before lecturing, find out what your client already knows. Before prescribing solutions, learn what your client has been considering or has already tried. Your turn to offer expertise isn't lost; it's just respectful and wise to honor the client's own knowledge and capability first. So what does this look like in practice?

The *How* of Offering Information and Advice
Asking Permission

One useful step is to ask permission before offering information or advice. If a client asks you for your advice, then you already have permission, though it's still wise to proceed cautiously.

CLIENT: Well what do you think I should do?

THERAPIST: I know some things that have worked for other people I've seen, but I'm interested in your own ideas as well. What thoughts do you have?

CLIENT: I'm not sure really. I guess I might ask some friends to support me as I go through this.

THERAPIST: The sounds like a good idea. What else?

CLIENT: Is there anything I could read?

THERAPIST: Well, there are several things I might suggest as possibilities. I don't know what would work best for you, but I can tell you a variety of options that other people have used successfully, if you'd like.

CLIENT: Yes, please!

hen a client hasn't already requested information or advice, you ı ask permission yourself:

- "Would it be all right if I suggest some things that have worked for other people?"
- "I can tell you some of the steps that people normally go through in making this kind of change. Would that be of interest?"
- "I wonder if I might explain a bit about. . . . "

ıost always, clients say "yes," and the act of having requested r permission honors their autonomy and can lower the shields of ·nsiveness.

oring Autonomy

ing permission honors self-direction. It's also possible to preface information or advice with language that further emphasizes the on's autonomy. In doing so, you are not really giving people any-g that they don't already have. You are only acknowledging the ı: the client's right to agree or disagree, to listen to or disregard t you say. In a sense you begin by yielding, by acknowledging truth, and in so doing make it more possible for clients to hear consider what you are offering (de Almeida Neto, 2017). Some ıples of such prefacing are:

- "I don't know whether this will make sense to you. . . . "
- "This may or may not apply in your own experience. . . . "
- "I wonder which of these options sounds most promising to you. . . . "
"This may or may not concern you, but there's something that worries me about this plan. Is it OK if I tell you what's bothering me?" (also asking permission)

In a way, you are offering permission to disregard or disagree wi
what you're about to say, simply acknowledging the freedom that c
ents already have. In interpersonal terms, you are removing yours
from a "one up" position, thereby making it more possible for t
client to hear what you want to say.

Choosing among Options

When offering advice on how to change, it's wise to offer seve
options rather than just one (Miller & Rollnick, 2013). Making o
suggestion at a time invites the client to tell you what's wrong w
that idea:

> CLIENT: Well, how do people quit drinking?
>
> THERAPIST: Some go to Alcoholics Anonymous meetings wh
> people in recovery support each other.
>
> CLIENT: No, I've tried that, and I didn't like it. Those people
> not like me.
>
> THERAPIST: There are some newer medications now to help p
> ple quit and decrease their craving for alcohol.
>
> CLIENT: I wouldn't want to depend on medications. It's li
> crutch.
>
> THERAPIST: Oh, well we have some group counseling here
> can help you learn skills for successful recovery.
>
> CLIENT: You know, I really don't like talking in groups. I
> uncomfortable.

Instead of making one suggestion, offer a variety of possible wa
proceed and ask clients to consider which might be best for them
mental set is different: to choose from among options rather tha
find fault with one possibility.

> THERAPIST: The good news is that most people do recover
> they do it in different ways. There is no one right appr
> for everybody. How about if I describe four or five diff
> possibilities that have worked for other people, and you
> sider which of these might best fit into your own life? W
> that be OK?

Ask-Provide-Ask

Avoid prolonged downloads of information. Instead, try offering any information in bite-sized chunks and checking in regularly. One rhythm for this is ask-provide-ask, using questions as bookends for the information you offer. Here are some kinds of opening questions before providing information:

- "Is it OK if I tell you a bit about _____?" (asking permission)
- "Tell me, what do you already know about _____?" (This avoids telling clients what they already know and allows you to respond to any misinformation.)
- "What would you most like to know about _____? What are you curious about?" (tailoring information to clients' interest)
- "Where would you like to start? What is most important to you?" (prioritizing)

Then after offering a bit of information, check in by asking your client to respond:

- "Does that make sense to you?"
- "What do you think about that?"
- "Is that something you have considered before?"
- "What more could I tell you about that?"

Then listen carefully to the client's answer. Ask-provide-ask is a single cycle, and soon this rhythm can become a conversational pattern of providing small bits of information interspersed with client responses and questions.

Listening

Empathic listening (Chapter 3) conveys respect and thereby further honors a person's individuality and autonomy. When you listen to your clients, they are more likely to listen to you. Respond with reflective listening to what they tell you and avoid getting into an argument about the information or their response. Empathic listening helps you make sure that you understand their responses and lets them know that you do.

THERAPIST: Does this surprise you, that people who have a high tolerance to alcohol are actually in greater danger?

CLIENT: I thought that if you can hold your liquor, it doesn't affect you as much.

THERAPIST: Yes, that sounds logical, and many people do believe that. You seem puzzled.

CLIENT: I just never thought much about it. I know that I can drink more than most people and not feel it.

THERAPIST: You know what your experience is, and haven't thought a lot about what it means. Actually, that kind of tolerance is risky. It's like not having a smoke alarm to warn you of harm. So, what are you thinking at this point?

CLIENT: Are you saying that I should cut down or quit?

THERAPIST: That's what I'm wondering. It's really up to you, of course, to decide what to do. What are you considering?

The language in this dialogue bespeaks a respectful partnership in which the client's own expertise matters as well as yours. After all, it really is the client who will decide what to do when it comes to behavior and lifestyle. Lecturing, warning, ordering, and arguing are unlikely to change behavior, and may well have the opposite effect of what you intend. Don't forget to listen well!

When you listen to your clients, they are more likely to listen to you.

Research on Offering Information and Advice

Whenever you give a client information that could be perceived as threatening, or offer advice for how she or he should change, you can anticipate a certain amount of reluctance, defensiveness, and inertia. Gerald Patterson and Marion Forgatch (1985) had therapists alternate their counseling style every 12 minutes, switching between periods of giving information and advice (teach/direct) and periods of reflective listening. Client resistance levels increased markedly during teach/direct segments and dropped when therapists were listening well. In a similar study (Glynn & Moyers, 2010), as counselors switched between 12-minute segments of behavioral analysis or person-centered motivational interviewing, clients systematically argued either against or for changing their alcohol use, respectively.

Nevertheless, professional advice does, on average, exert a small positive effect on behavior change. This has been most extensively studied in advice to quit smoking (Aveyard et al., 2012; Stead et al., 2013) or reduce heavy drinking (DiClemente, Corno, Graydon, Wiprovnick, & Knoblach, 2017; Lenz, Rosenbaum, & Sheperis, 2016; McQueen, Howe, Allan, Mains, & Hardy, 2011; Moyer, Finney, Swearingen, & Vergun, 2002; Samson & Tanner-Smith, 2015; Smedslund et al., 2011; Vasilaki, Hosier, & Cox, 2006). Professional advice has also been associated with positive change in depression (McNaughton, 2009; Schmidt & Miller, 1983) and physical activity (Vijay et al., 2016). Average effect sizes of professional advice are modest (0.2 to 0.3) but significant.

As emphasized throughout this book, it matters *how* you advise. To begin with, information and advice are not separate from, but should be offered within, the context of the interpersonal skills described in previous chapters. In essence, the goal is to offer any advice or information within a relational context that makes it safer for clients to receive and consider. What is important is not just the content of what you offer, but also how and when you say it.

A review of effective advice interventions for harmful alcohol use identified six elements that were often present, abbreviated in the acronym FRAMES (Bien, Miller, & Tonigan, 1993; Miller & Sanchez, 1994). Clients were often provided with individual Feedback (such as test results) regarding their drinking and its consequences. Strong emphasis was placed on personal Responsibility for change, meaning that it was the clients' own free choice. "The manner in which such advice is given should reinforce a sense of autonomy and self-direction" (G. Edwards & Orford, 1977, p. 346). Nevertheless, the professional helpers did offer Advice to make a change. Rather than prescribing a single solution, clients were often offered a Menu of approaches from which to choose, again emphasizing autonomous choice. Whenever the style of counseling was described, it was Empathic, a person-centered reflective listening style (Chapter 3). Finally, effective brief interventions also supported Self-efficacy, optimism that the client was capable of making change (Chapter 8).

Thus, advice was offered within the context of empathic listening, empowerment, and honoring autonomy.

KEY POINTS

- Providing information and advice is a normal part of helping roles.
- Providing professional advice has a small positive effect, on average, and varies with how you advise.
- The professional style of guiding represents a balance between listening to clients and offering information and advice.
- Psychological reactance is the well-documented tendency for people to act contrary to recommendations from others, even when they agree with the advice.
- Effective brief interventions often include FRAMES: Feedback, Responsibility, Advice, Menu of options, Empathic style, and Support for self-efficacy.
- Asking permission, honoring autonomy, listening, and offering choices can help clients to hear and consider your advice.

CHAPTER 11

The Far Side of Complexity

In the preceding chapters, we have been journeying through considerable complexity as to what makes a helper more effective. The evidence-based factors described in this book include empathy, acceptance, positive regard, genuineness, focus, hope, evocation, and offering information and advice. A reasonable case can be made that each of these therapeutic skills contributes to more effective helping relationships.

At this point, you may be wondering how any therapist could possibly be proficient in all or even a few of these valuable skills. How is a clinician supposed to become more empathic *and* accepting *and* genuine *and* graceful in giving advice, all in one career?

Yet, surely there is some overlap among these relational factors, just as evidence-based treatment techniques may reduce to a smaller number of higher-order processes of change (Prochaska, 1994; Prochaska & DiClemente, 1984). Similarly, symptoms of what seem to be separate disorders such as anxiety and depression may reflect a superordinate form like neuroticism (Barlow et al., 2014), and be treatable with interventions tailored to that construct (Barlow, Sauer-Zavala, Carl, Bullis, & Ellard, 2017). Just as with disorders and treatments, interpersonal skills appear to be different and yet may have a higher-order structure. Counselors who are skilled in accurate empathy are more likely to communicate warmth and acceptance. Teachers who regularly affirm students' strengths probably also convey greater hopefulness about their success. Carl Rogers and his students highlighted three of the above as interrelated core conditions for effective counseling: accurate empathy, positive regard, and genuineness (Rogers, 1959; Rogers et al., 1967; Truax & Carkhuff, 1967). Even relatively brief exposure to helpers who are high in these therapeutic factors may be enough to foster positive change in some long-standing problems (Babor, 2004; Bernstein et al., 2005; Gaume, Gmel, Faouzi, & Daeppen, 2009; Miller, 2000).

Is there a higher-order level of healers' helpfulness? Toward the end of his life, Rogers was writing about *presence* as a foundational state of consciousness, a way of being from which acceptance, empathy, and genuineness flow naturally (Rogers, 1980c, 1980d; Weinraub, 2018). Not a religious man, Rogers nevertheless described the experience as if "my inner spirit has reached out and touched the inner spirit of the other . . . and becomes a part of something larger." He likened it to mystical experiences of unity and confessed, "I am compelled to believe that I, like many others, have underestimated the importance of this mystical, spiritual dimension," averring, "here many readers, I am sure, will part company with me" (Rogers, 1980d, pp. 129–130).

> Even brief exposure to helpers who are high in accurate empathy, positive regard, and genuineness can foster positive change.

Such experiences fascinated William James (1994/1902) at a time when psychology had not grown far from its historic roots in philosophy. By the mid-20th century, however, the discipline of psychology had distanced itself from, even developed an aversion to, religious discourse (Miller, 2005), with the notable exception of the relatively isolated specialization in psychology of religion (Hood, Hill, & Spilka, 2018). With a dominance of logical positivism, academic psychology first lost its soul (the Greek root *psyche* of "psychology") and then its mind (Delaney & DiClemente, 2005), although considerable progress was made in regaining the mind through studies of cognition and consciousness. By the end of the century, *psyche* was back as well. The door had reopened to the topic of spirituality, reflected in the first books published on the subject by the American Psychological Association (Miller, 1999; Richards & Bergin, 1997; Shafranske, 1996). As a profession, American psychologists remain far less religious than their clients, but do clearly affirm spirituality as important in their lives (Delaney, Miller, & Bisonó, 2007). Interest has also grown in understanding character and virtues (Peterson & Seligman, 2004) and in the ancient meditative discipline of mindfulness (K. W. Brown, Ryan, & Creswell, 2007; S. C. Hayes et al., 2011), which Shari Geller and Leslie Greenberg (2018) have linked to Rogers's concept of therapeutic presence.

One can (though need not) appeal to transpersonal roots in order to conceptualize higher-order states of consciousness and behavior. Ancient writings describe benevolent master virtues such as *mettā* ("benevolence") in Buddhism and *rahmah* ("compassion") in Islam. First-century Christian writings described *agape* in behavioral terms as a selfless form of loving that is patient and kind, and does not insist on its own way. The still older Hebrew concept of *hesed* was so multifaceted that the 16th-century translator Myles Coverdale despaired of finding a single word to adequately render it in English, so he created a new term by combining two other words: "loving" and "kindness." "Lovingkindness" encompasses both compassionate intention (loving) and its benevolent enactment (kindness). Drawing on these ancient descriptions of such master virtues, William Miller (2017) described lovingkindness as encompassing a dozen behavioral virtues: compassion, empathy, contentment, generosity, hope, affirmation, forgiveness, patience, humility, gratitude, helpfulness, and yielding. This list obviously overlaps with the attributes of effective helpers described in this volume and may suggest some additional potential therapeutic factors to explore. Obviously, such lovingkindness can be manifest in all manner of relationships, not merely in helping or therapeutic professions.

Lovingkindness encompasses both compassionate intention and its benevolent enactment.

Is there resonance between higher-order virtues like lovingkindness or *mettā* and the therapeutic factors that characterize effective helpers? Justice Oliver Wendell Holmes Jr. is quoted as saying, "I would not give a fig for the simplicity this side of complexity, but I would give my life for the simplicity on the other side of complexity." Indeed, it does not work well to begin with simplicity. Telling therapists to "just love your clients" is unlikely to be helpful, in part because "love" has so many possible meanings. C. S. Lewis (1960), for example, described four types of love that were differentiated in ancient Greek, three of which are relationships best avoided with clients: erotic love, familial love, and sentimental attraction. It is the fourth type of love, *agape,* that describes selfless and active commitment to another's happiness, well-being, and freedom from suffering (Fromm, 1956; Lewis, 1960; Miller, 2000).

Early in the development of motivational interviewing, Miller and Rollnick discovered the importance of a higher-order understanding. Soon after the publication of their first edition (Miller & Rollnick, 1991), they observed trainees practicing the techniques they had taught and were dismayed. It was as if the trainees were trying to use techniques "on" clients, to outsmart or manipulate them into changing. It was not the trainees' fault. Obviously, their training had left out something vital, but what was it? The missing piece, they discovered, was the underlying mindset or "heartset" with which one practices. They began calling this the underlying spirit of motivational interviewing, encompassing partnership, acceptance, compassion, and evocation (Miller & Rollnick, 2013; Rollnick & Miller, 1995). There is an obvious kinship to what Rogers described as the clinician's attitudes that underlie and inspire practice, and his concern that a person-centered approach should not be reduced to a set of techniques.

So, what simplicity lies on the far side of complexity in therapeutic relationships? It has been described as a way of being (Rogers, 1980d), a higher-order consciousness and practice variously called presence (Geller & Greenberg, 2018; Weinraub, 2018), responsiveness (Norcross, 2011), real relationship (Gelso et al., 2018), compassion (Armstrong, 2010; Rakel, 2018; The Dalai Lama & Vreeland, 2001), or lovingkindness (Fromm, 1956; Salzberg, 1995; R. Shapiro, 2006). If attaining such perfected simplicity were a prerequisite for engaging in helping relationships, then no one could begin. Like musical virtuosity, there is some component of preparedness or talent, but proficiency is also actualized over time through deliberate practice (Chow et al., 2015; Ericsson, Krampe, & Tesch-Römer, 1993; Ericsson & Pool, 2016; Gladwell, 2008). As Shakespeare's Hamlet advised in Elizabethan English:

> Assume a virtue, if you have it not.
> That monster, custom, . . . is angel yet in this,
> That to the use of actions fair and good
> He likewise gives a [garment],

> That aptly is put on. . . .
> For use almost can change the stamp of nature.
> (*Hamlet*, Act 3, Scene 4)

The good news, then, is that the interpersonal skills described in this book may, with intentional practice, become second-nature habits. Some individuals have a head start in interpersonal talent. There are people who seem to affirm or reflect as naturally as breathing. Some readily communicate acceptance and hope to those who are fortunate to be their friends or clients. There are teachers who, with genuine presence, find and evoke the best in their students. Such skills are not present at birth, but emerge through a combination of talent and practice.

Perhaps simplicity lies on the far side of complexity because it represents a *confluence* of the individual streams that we have been considering in this volume. The streams may or may not flow from a single source, but can converge over time. The deliberate practice of a particular interpersonal skill not only facilitates a certain freedom or ease in its use, but begins to change one's nature as well. Faithfully practicing several such skills can have a synergistic effect at a level often described as virtue or character (Brooks, 2015; Franklin, 2012/1785; Peterson & Seligman, 2004). Rogers described the confluence of accurate empathy, unconditional positive regard, and congruence as a "way of being" and therapeutic presence (Rogers, 1980d; Weinraub, 2018).

Like many truths, this therapeutic presence, this simplicity beyond complexity, is somewhat paradoxical. It is at once both behavioral practice and underlying attitude or spirit, and the two sculpt each other. Faithful practice strengthens the guiding value system that, in turn, is expressed in practice. Benjamin Franklin (1785) reflected on this cumulative emergence of values:

> We stand at the crossroads, each minute, each hour, each day, making choices. We choose the thoughts we allow ourselves to think, the passions we allow ourselves to feel, and the actions we allow ourselves to perform. Each choice is made in the context of whatever value system we have selected to govern our lives. In selecting that value system, we are, in a very real way, making the most important choice we will ever make.

Clinical training is clearly meant to inform and develop practice behavior in a way that benefits those being served. What has received little scientific attention is how clinical training and practice also shape the values and character of practitioners themselves. We have sometimes mused that participants in clinical training should first sign a statement of informed consent, that practicing what we preach may change them. We do believe, for example, that acceptance and empathic understanding, when practiced over time, can render one a more accepting, patient, and compassionate person. Perhaps this is the very simplicity that lies beyond the complexity of practice with which we have wrestled through the foregoing chapters.

How do clinical training and practice shape the values and character of practitioners?

KEY POINTS

- The therapeutic skills described in this book are not separate, but overlap and are intertwined.
- These skills resemble and enact some long-honored human virtues.
- In their confluence, these complex therapeutic skills may over time become a simpler way of being.

PART III

LEARNING, TRAINING, AND CLINICAL SCIENCE

If therapists don't automatically get better with practice, what can be done to develop your own therapeutic skills or to help others do so? In this closing section, we consider first how you might improve your own clinical expertise and your clients' outcomes (Chapter 12). Next, we discuss implications of the knowledge presented in the foregoing chapters for clinical training, supervision, and coaching (Chapter 13). Finally in Chapter 14, we step back to take a broader view still, wondering what the lessons of these decades of work may suggest for the enterprise of clinical science.

Developing Expertise

Why did you choose a helping profession as a career path? Most therapists hope to reduce suffering and promote positive growth in the people they serve, but what if you can't really tell whether your work is making a difference?

The profession of counseling and psychotherapy suffers from some unique but surmountable obstacles to developing expertise. Nowhere is this more apparent than in the widely replicated finding that therapists' years of experience are unrelated to their actual expertise, interpersonal skills, ability to form therapeutic alliance, or client outcomes (e.g., Goldberg et al., 2016; Hersoug, Hoglend, Monsen, & Havik, 2001; Lafferty et al., 1989; Truax & Carkhuff, 1976; Tracey, Wampold, Lichtenberg, & Goodyear, 2014; Witteman, Weiss, & Metzmacher, 2012). On average, counselors and psychotherapists don't automatically get better with practice! When a relationship *is* observed between experience and skill, it may not even be in the hoped for direction (Erekson et al., 2017). More experienced psychotherapists can be *less* likely to have favorable outcomes than newer therapists do (Goldberg, Hoyt, Nissen-Lie, Nielsen, & Wampold, 2018; Hersoug et al., 2001).

In many professions, experience is a desirable attribute because it offers the promise of increased skills and better outcomes. Surgeons, for example, usually get better with practice. A surgeon who has done a thousand procedures is more skillful than the resident doing his or her first. Rates of patient mortality, complications, and adverse outcomes decrease with surgeons' experience, a phenomenon known as the "surgeon volume effect" (Morche, Mathes, & Pieper, 2016; Mowat, Maher, & Ballard, 2016).

What accounts for this difference between surgeons and psychotherapists? There is clear and immediate feedback about success during and after surgery. Complications are apparent and outcomes are seen relatively quickly. Furthermore, surgeons seldom work alone. There are colleagues present so that procedures are observed and may be video-recorded for later review.

Counselors and psychotherapists don't automatically get better with practice.

Lack of reliable feedback is an occupational hazard in counseling and psychotherapy. Treatment sessions usually happen unobserved behind closed doors, with no record other than the therapist's own notes. Behavioral health outcomes are commonly judged by how well clients are doing after treatment has ended, and if practitioners receive any information at all about their clients' outcomes, the feedback is long delayed. Twenty years of practice in a feedback vacuum are unlikely to yield much improvement in a complex skill.

So, if experience in itself does not lead to increased expertise, how can you improve your interpersonal skills and other elements of your practice that produce better client outcomes? Barriers to learning may reside at a systemic and policy level. Yet, there are things you can do to develop your own expertise that are entirely within your purview, and that indeed may not be achievable by any other means. That is the focus of this chapter: what you as an individual practitioner can do to get better at what you do, even in challenging work settings. We will consider possible systemic changes in Chapter 13.

Deliberate Practice

Suppose you want to hone your golf skills. You plan to practice driving, so you head to the golf course with your clubs and pay for a large bucket of balls. Just as you arrive at the practice range, a thick fog rolls in. Every time you hit a ball, it disappears into the fog within a few feet, gone from sight. Maybe it felt pretty good, but you can't tell where the ball went. Will your drive improve much?

Similarly, students in our introductory psychology course have the option of taking online practice quizzes in preparation for exams, receiving immediate feedback of the correct answers. This can dramatically improve their performance on future exams. However, if they were to answer 500 practice items but receive no feedback (or inaccurate feedback) about whether their answers were correct, it would be unlikely to help them score better in the future.

That is the predicament for most practitioners who would like to develop expertise in delivering therapeutic interventions. You receive some initial training, accept a job, and become absorbed in clinical service. Your work is demanding, unremitting, and draws on your capacity for compassion. There is little time to observe other therapists or receive coaching on your own skills. The supervision that you do receive tends to focus on administrative concerns and the management of high-risk situations. You may see many cases but rarely learn how your clients fare once treatment is over. Through anecdotal feedback you may occasionally hear about some good (or more often, poor) outcomes. Decades can go by without much reliable feedback about how effective your work has been.

Early in my career, I (WRM) was assigned to do intake interviews with whoever walked through the door of a large behavioral health facility for veterans. It was fascinating work. I got to see a huge variety of people with a rich panoply of presenting concerns. I developed tentative diagnoses, wrote reports, and referred the veterans to one of dozens of service units within the hospital. After a few months, however, I realized that I could do this for the rest of my life and not get any better at my work. I never found out whether my provisional diagnoses were confirmed, or even if the people ever arrived at the service to which I had referred them.

Working in the dark can stunt your professional growth and lead to burnout. One remedy is to invest some time in "deliberate practice," a term borrowed from professional expertise research in fields as diverse as medicine, sports, music, chess, and business (Ericsson et al., 1993; Ericsson & Pool, 2016). Time spent in deliberate practice distinguishes clinicians with the best client outcomes from those with the worst (Chow et al., 2015).

Deliberate practice in counseling and psychotherapy involves two critical components. First,

> *Working in the dark can stunt your professional growth and lead to burnout.*

you intentionally engage in activities designed to improve specific aspects of your work through repetition and successive refinement. Second, you receive reliable feedback about your practice (e.g., Westra et al., 2020). In this formula (see Figure 12.1), if either of these two elements is zero, then the total (i.e., the increase in your expertise) will also be zero. As a simple example, basketball players regularly practice specific skills. When practicing foul shots, the feedback is immediate: Either the ball goes in or it doesn't. Such immediate and binary feedback is optimal for learning, though seldom available in the practice of counseling and psychotherapy. Of course, therapy outcomes are more complex than foul shots, but the analogy still holds: Without feedback, proficiency is unlikely to improve.

Deliberate practice can be used to develop anything from clinical microskills to macro-applications in actual practice. Drawing again on a basketball analogy, microskills for deliberate practice might be foul shots, dribbling, passing, and lay-ups. Complexity comes in combining these at a macro level in practice sessions, pick-up games, or actual competition. The most basic prerequisite for developing clinical skills is to set aside time for engaging in deliberate practice (S. D. Miller, Hubble, & Chow, 2020). Where does this time come from? As with musicians, athletes, artists, and other professionals, it must come from other areas of your work or life. Beyond devoting time for deliberate practice, it is also important to have a way to record your practice so that it can be reviewed by yourself or others.

There are at least three broad domains of therapeutic expertise: conceptual formulation, technical aspects of specific treatments, and interpersonal skills. Examples of conceptual formulation skills include clinical evaluation, differential diagnosis, selecting interventions among evidence-based options, and deciding when to include other members of a client's social network in treatment.

Technical skills focus on the particular aspects of treatments that require specialized knowledge and expertise. Most treatments include elements related to the presumed mechanisms of efficacy; for example, conditioning or counterconditioning, biofeedback, transference, cognitive schemas, or behavioral coping skills. To provide such treatments with fidelity requires competent delivery of these specific components (Bellg et al., 2004; Fixsen, Blase, & Van Dyke, 2019; Henggeler, Schoenwald, Letourneau, & Edwards, 2002; Miller &

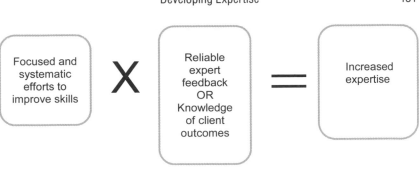

FIGURE 12.1. Formula for Deliberate Practice.

Rollnick, 2014). A common aid for learning and practicing technical skills is a detailed therapist manual or protocol offering step-by-step instructions, sometimes accompanied by checklists for clinicians or observers to use in documenting fidelity.

As discussed in previous chapters, the therapist's repertoire of interpersonal therapeutic skills is an important evidence-based component of competence and outcomes in counseling and psychotherapy (e.g., Barnicot et al., 2014; Zuroff et al., 2010). In this chapter, we focus on developing expertise in this third element of competence in counseling: interpersonal therapeutic skills. We begin by discussing *what* to practice, before moving on to six possible sources of feedback to support your learning.

Interpersonal Microskills

A useful approach to gaining mastery as a therapist is to practice specific interpersonal microskills before integrating them into complex practice (Carkhuff, 2019; Egan, 2014). Pianists practice scales, paramedics learn cardiopulmonary resuscitation procedures, tennis players drill forehand and backhand strokes until they become comfortable, even automatic.

As an example, we will focus on the microskill of reflective listening (Chapter 3). The technique is not the entire skill; just as jazz is more than playing scales, accurate empathy is more than offering reflections (Bozarth, 1984; Rogers, 1980b), but it's a good beginning.

A first step is to understand and recognize what empathic listening statements are. Can you pick them out in a transcript or recording of a counseling session? Various observational systems are available that define therapist reflections (Lane et al., 2005; Miller, Hedrick, & Orlofsky, 1991; Moyers, Rowell, et al., 2016) and other behavioral aspects of empathy (Campinez Navarro et al., 2016). You can use an observational code to identify empathic listening statements and differentiate them from other kinds of therapist responses, perhaps comparing your results with expert or colleagues' coding.

As a simple example, here is a transcribed excerpt from an initial interview with a woman referred by her doctor (Miller, Rollnick, & Moyers, 2013). The only therapist responses coded here are questions and reflections.

THERAPIST: When you called, you said that your doctor had asked you to come and talk with me, and he did send me a message just indicating you'd be coming. So, fill me in a little bit. Tell me how you've been feeling and what's been happening. — *Open question*

CLIENT: I've just been really tired lately. I don't feel like I have enough energy to do the things I need to do during the day.

THERAPIST: Like the battery's running low. — *Reflection—a metaphor*

CLIENT: Yeah.

THERAPIST: Sleepy. — *Reflection—a guess*

CLIENT: Yeah. I'm not really sleeping well either.

THERAPIST: Tell me a bit about that. What's happening with sleep? — *Open question*

CLIENT: Well, I go to bed at the same time every night, but instead of sleeping through the night, I'll get up at 3:30 in the morning almost every day, and then I can't really fall back to sleep.

THERAPIST: So, that's not normal for you. You're used to sleeping pretty well through the night, and now you're finding you're waking up in the middle of the night, and not getting back to sleep.

Reflection

CLIENT: Right.

THERAPIST: OK. What else has been happening?

Open question

CLIENT: I don't know. I mean, I went to the doctor because I was just really tired, you know, so I'm not really sure.

THERAPIST: You were getting checked out just to see if there was something physically wrong.

Reflection

CLIENT: Yes.

THERAPIST: And what did your doctor say?

Open question

CLIENT: He asked me if I might be depressed.

THERAPIST: What do you think?

Open question

CLIENT: I don't know. I mean, I don't have that much experience with it.

THERAPIST: What do you know about depression?

Open question to learn what she already knows before providing information

CLIENT: I don't know. I guess it seems like a lot of people take medication for it these days.

This is just an example of how recorded sessions can be reviewed for the presence of particular therapist responses—in this case, questions and reflections.

After being able to recognize reflections, a second step is to practice generating reflective listening statements yourself. This can be done in response to a written or recorded list of sample client statements (Truax & Carkhuff, 1967, 1976). Alone or with others, listen to a clinical session, stopping regularly after client statements to generate possible empathic responses. When reflections are spoken aloud, you can also practice the "music" as well as the words—for example, turning your voice down at the end to form a statement rather than a question.

As generating single reflections becomes easier, try it live in nonclinical conversations. A colleague could role-play a client, but we find it is better to use "real play" in which the speaker talks about his or her own experience. The listener's role is to respond exclusively or primarily with reflective listening statements (Miller, 2018; Rosengren, 2018). You can also try including reflective listening in your everyday conversations.

Finally, try it in clinical practice. Here, it is particularly useful to have a recording (with client permission) that you can review later. At moments where you might ordinarily ask a question or offer advice, try reflective listening instead. When attempting a new skill, begin with a few less difficult cases, working up to application in other more challenging cases (Love, Kilmer, & Callahan, 2016). Using plenty of reflections to balance the questions you ask might be a particularly important skill to start with, because it predicts better client outcomes (DeVargas & Stormshak, 2020).

The above description illustrates a full continuum of deliberate practice, from recognition, to generating individual therapeutic responses, to conversational practice in nonclinical and clinical contexts. The same successive steps can be used in practicing other therapeutic interpersonal skills described in prior chapters.

Sources of Feedback

Reliable feedback is a prerequisite for learning. Without it, you're golfing in the fog. A lack of reliable and timely information about client outcomes is a likely explanation of why counselors and psychotherapists do not develop the kind of progressive expertise that characterizes other professions (Tracey et al., 2014).

Feedback alone is not enough, of course. Extensive and accurate feedback is of little use if you don't adjust your practice behavior

accordingly. A common finding
after clinical workshop training,
even when it includes experien-

> *Reliable feedback is a
> prerequisite for learning.*

tial rehearsal, is that therapists quickly return to prior practice habits, yet believe they are now using the new skills (Fixsen, Naoom, Blase, Friedman, & Wallace, 2005; Miller & Mount, 2001; Miller, Sorensen, Selzer, & Brigham, 2006).

Next, we consider six possible sources of feedback on practice. They vary in simplicity and in the delay between practice and feedback. They can also vary in reliability and validity. Some kinds of feedback may be irrelevant or even antithetical to good client outcomes, a consideration that we address in the next section of this chapter. We begin here with sources of feedback that are most proximal—closest to actual practice behavior—and then move on to those that are more distal or delayed. The first two can be done on your own as reflective practice, whereas the remainder involve receiving feedback from others.

Client In-Session Responses

An ideal form of feedback occurs immediately after a practiced skill, much like the golfer's ball going into the cup. Here, you are observing how a client responds immediately to your in-session behavior. For example, when you offer an empathic listening statement (Chapter 3), you normally receive immediate client feedback about its accuracy. Similarly, a psychodynamic clinician who provides an interpretation observes carefully how the client responds, offering information about whether it was apt or premature.

In Chapter 9 on evocation, we discussed some in-session client responses that presage better outcomes. Within client-centered counseling, for example, the practitioner attends to clients' in-session depth of experiencing that is associated with positive growth (Hill, 1990; Luborsky et al., 1971; Orlinsky & Howard, 1986; Pascuel-Leone & Yervomenko, 2017; Watson & Bedard, 2006; Wiser & Goldfried, 1998). In motivational interviewing, the clinician notices and seeks to evoke client change talk, relative to the amount of sustain talk (Apodaca et al., 2016; Drage et al., 2019; Gaume et al., 2010; Moyers et al., 2009). Various technical and relational skills can be tried to facilitate these client processes. The immediate in-session feedback tells you which practice behaviors increase (or decrease) the outcome-relevant client responses. In other words, you can try various in-session methods and get immediate feedback about whether the relevant client response occurs.

Similarly, some in-session responses signal poorer outcomes if unaddressed. Change is less likely to occur to the extent that a client argues against it (M. Magill et al., 2018; Miller & Rose, 2009; Vader et al., 2010). Other forms of "resistance" or discord in the working alliance are evoked by particular practice behaviors and signal a poorer outcome (Bischoff & Tracey, 1995; Drage et al., 2019; Klonek et al., 2014; Patterson & Chamberlain, 1994). Thus, the occurrence of resistant behavior in a treatment session could be regarded as a signal not to repeat whatever was eliciting the resistance, and to try other responses to alleviate it (Engle & Arkowitz, 2006; Miller & Rollnick, 2013). Deliberate practice in responding to client resistance can both increase clinician skill (Westra et al., in press) and decrease subsequent client-resistant responses (Di Bartolomeo, Shukla, Westra, Ghashghaei, & Olson, in press).

If particular client in-session responses are reliably related to outcome, then observant therapists can receive ongoing feedback about what practice behaviors increase or decrease these responses. When feedback immediately follows therapist behavior, it is more likely to shape future practice.

Self-Review of Practice

A second strategy for reflective practice is audio or video recordings of your work (with client permission) for later reflective review (Raingruber, 2003). The recording of service transactions is now commonplace, and we find that clients rarely object when it is presented as routine with the purpose of improving the quality of service. Be clear with clients about how confidentiality will be protected, how long a recording will be retained, who (if anyone besides yourself) will observe it, and when and how it will be destroyed afterward. A signed consent for such recording is appropriate. We also tell clients that the recording can be turned off at any time during a session if there is material they do not wish to have recorded—a protection that most clients appreciate but rarely invoke.

We continue to be impressed with how much more we can hear when reviewing a session afterward, things that we may have missed while in the midst of it. If listening for particular kinds of client speech, for example, it is often easier to notice it on a second hearing. You can also go back and listen to your own responses that preceded or followed specific client responses. What did you do that evoked client change talk or experiencing? If your client became defensive or argumentative, or just seemed to shut down for a bit, what were you doing just before that? In one study, clinician-reported deliberate practices that were most related to superior client outcomes included reviewing difficult/challenging cases alone, mentally running through and reflecting on past sessions, and mentally running through and reflecting on what to do in future sessions (Chow et al., 2015).

You can also just focus on your own responses. When trying to improve your ratio of reflections to questions (Chapter 3), you can literally count them, consider how many of your reflections were complex versus simple, and what proportion of your questions were open or closed. You can hear the music of speech in a way that may evade you during a session. At the end of reflections, did you inflect your voice upward or downward, and how did clients respond to each? Just as athletes carefully review their game-day films, you can learn a lot by focusing on the fine-grained details of your sessions.

There are observation codes that you can use to structure your reflective practice. They vary in complexity from simple response counts to systems that assign codes to every therapist and client response. When using such codes in self-review of practice, we recommend using counts of specific responses, because it is difficult to be reliable and objective in making global ratings of your own work. As an example, therapists are much more accurate at identifying when they have offered a reflection versus a question than they are at evaluating their level of overall empathy. Global constructs such as genuineness, empathy, and positive regard suffer from a tendency toward self-evaluation bias (i.e., people tend to rate themselves more favorably on these constructs than an objective observer would). On global ratings, therapists rarely evaluate their own "level" correctly, as compared with expert coder/observers.

Self-review of practice may feel safer than allowing others to hear and respond to your work, but it also has serious limitations. Imagine trying to learn tennis, piano, chess, gymnastics, or surgery all by yourself. Yes, you can read books and practice specific techniques until they become more consistent and comfortable. An experienced coach, however, will often observe things that you miss and

Self-review of practice has serious limitations.

can make specific, important, and sometimes simple suggestions to improve your expertise.

Expert Feedback and Coaching

A common strategy in learning any complex skill is to work with a coach who has more expertise than you do. Who might be able to help you develop specific technical or relational skills that will actually improve your clients' outcomes?

When a coach observes your practice, you can receive timely feedback. We learned early in our teaching careers that when novice therapists emerged from a treatment session to tell us what had happened, our ability to help them was limited. Often what was important is what the therapist did *not* notice. Consequently, we have supervised through direct observation, first via one-way mirrors (e.g., Miller et al., 1980), and then via video or audio recordings of sessions. Direct observation can be intimidating in initial training, but one never says to a tennis coach, "Don't watch me," or to a piano teacher, "Don't listen to me. I'd be too embarrassed!" In fact, coaching via observation is a rich opportunity for learning, and one that too often disappears after completing a graduate degree.

Coaches can also provide prompt feedback with simulated practice, as in interviewing a "standard patient" played by a trained actor. Professional actors often do not respond quite like actual clients do, especially when therapists exhibit advanced skills (Decker, Carroll, Nich, Canning-Ball, & Martino, 2013). Nevertheless, such simulations do provide a reliable sample of baseline professional expertise and an opportunity to improve it (Miller & Mount, 2001; Miller, Yahne, Moyers, Martinez, & Pirritano, 2004; Sacco et al., 2017). As mentioned above, it is also possible to practice skills such as accurate empathy (Chapter 3) in "real-play" conversations where people being interviewed are not pretending to be someone else, but are talking about experiences in their own lives (Miller, Moyers, et al., 2005).

The usefulness of expert feedback depends, of course, on the validity of the coach's advice, remembering that years of experience alone do not improve clinical practice. As with clinicians themselves, supervisors or coaches may focus on aspects of practice that are unrelated or even detrimental to client outcomes. Expert advice is best supplemented by structured observational codes and objective forms of outcome monitoring.

Working Alliance

There is a reliable relationship between clients' ratings of working alliance (WA)—how well they and their therapist are working together—and their eventual treatment outcomes (van Bentham et al., in press). Ratings of WA are therefore a reasonable proxy for treatment effectiveness. Here, then, is another opportunity for feedback to improve your professional expertise (Ackerman & Hilsenroth, 2003; Owen, Miller, Seidel, & Chow, 2016). WA is best when the therapist and client agree about what they are trying to accomplish, have a strong emotional bond, and are collaborating to accomplish the goals they have set together. In many ways, a good WA is like two people in a canoe, using their paddles in synchrony to get from one side of a lake to the other. WA involves not only developing interpersonal skills, but also adjusting those skills flexibly in response to clients' unique needs. A commonly used WA measure is the Working Alliance Inventory, which has separate versions for clients, therapists, and observers, and is available at *https://wai.profhorvath.com/ Downloads*.

As with any human relationship, disruptions in WA can and do occur (Safran et al., 1990). This may happen, for example, when there is a disagreement about the goals of treatment, or when the therapist and client experience discord or are not cooperating to pull their oars in the same direction (Safran & Muran, 2000). Paying careful attention to the working relationship you have with your client is important because ruptures in WA are consistently associated with poorer client outcomes (Eubanks, Muran, & Safran, 2018). Alliance-focused therapy (AFT; Eubanks-Carter, Muran, & Safran, 2015) was developed to help therapists recognize and resolve ruptures in WA, independent of whatever treatment method is being used. AFT is meant to strengthen clinicians' ability to recognize and tolerate their own difficult emotions (such as anxiety) or hostility from their clients by increasing their self-awareness, affect regulation, and interpersonal sensitivity. This approach focuses on a here-and-now orientation, often engaging the client in improving the therapeutic relationship as a joint endeavor. AFT has been operationalized in a treatment manual (Eubanks-Carter et al., 2015), evaluated in randomized clinical trials, and added to other treatments (e.g., cognitive-behavioral treatments) to improve outcomes (Muran et al., 2018). AFT stems from a psychodynamic tradition, but is compatible as an addition to other forms of counseling and psychotherapy (Muran et al., 2018; Safran et al., 2014).

Collaborative Community of Practice

What if you don't have regular access to an expert coach? An alternative is to form a collaborative community of practice, a learning group whose sole purpose is to help you get better at what you do. It is not for competition or evaluation, but for honing skills together through deliberate practice in a group setting. A learning community can include people with differing levels of current skill. It is not for talking *about* skills, but for actually practicing them.

In structuring a community of practice, we recommend a solid foundation in positive affirmation of good practice. It is easy to criticize. We might be able to list 14 things that a learner could do better, but if we do so, nothing is likely to change except the learner's morale. When observing skills, whether in a recording or in live practice, what is the person doing *well*? Then within the context of affirming what is already good practice, perhaps make one suggestion for what the learner could try next. This requires discerning, among all the suggestions that could be made, what is one good next step in this person's learning.

Here is a specific group format that we developed for a community of practice with up to 12 participants. It requires two dice. We have everyone count off and remember their number. One person at a time offers practice to be observed. It might be part of a recorded session, or a live role-play or real-play practice with another group member serving as the "client" or speaker. We place a 10-minute limit on observed practice as a balance between what is enough time to get a good work sample, and what can become boring or wearing. Except for the practitioner being observed, everyone else has two tasks: (1) to notice what the counselor is doing well, taking notes on specific examples of good practice, and (2) to decide what *one* suggestion they would make for the counselor to try next in developing expertise. At the end of the 10-minute sample, there is an affirmation round in which observers take turns commenting on what they noticed as good practice, giving specific examples whenever possible. Each person makes a single such comment (and only one); then after all have spoken, the members can continue to offer their observations of good practice until everything on everyone's lists has been mentioned. Now the count-off numbers become important. The person who is receiving feedback rolls a die (if there are 6 people or fewer in the group) or two dice (if 7–12 people). The individual whose number comes up gets to offer his or her *one* suggestion. And that's it. No one else offers a suggestion no matter how brilliant it may be. Then it's time for another round.

The randomness in selecting who will offer the feedback is important—that is the purpose of rolling the dice (or some other source of randomness). We have found that the person who most *wants* to offer feedback is not always the best participant to do so. Randomness further requires every observer to actively think about what one suggestion he or she might offer.

As with self-review of practice, a totally self-contained community of practice has a shortcoming. Peer learning communities are not substitutes for expert feedback, and when used as the only strategy for learning therapeutic skills, they may promote unwarranted confidence, as is common when therapists evaluate their own skills (Herschell, Kolko, Baumann, & Davis, 2010). Nevertheless, peer learning can have a powerful and unique impact. Think of the study groups that enthusiastic college students form outside their most difficult classes. They are not intended to replace the professor's feedback and knowledge, but they do encourage active learning in a way that enlivens and enriches the formal instruction they receive.

Outcome Monitoring

A sixth potential source of feedback is to monitor outcomes for everyone you have treated, or at least a representative sample of clients. This is routine in treatment outcome research, where all treated participants are followed over time. Whereas outcome information tends to be sporadic and anecdotal in most clinical practices, clinical trials seek to document the outcomes of all "intent to treat" participants. Although outcomes *during* treatment are of primary interest in pharmaceutical trials (Miller, LoCastro, Longabaugh, O'Malley, & Zweben, 2005), psychotherapy is often judged by the maintenance of gains and quality of life after treatment has ended (Longabaugh, Mattson, Connors, & Cooney, 1994; Miller, Walters, et al., 2001). Consequently, the results of behavioral treatment trials tend to be revealed well after therapy is over, a substantial delay between practice and feedback.

How might you learn about your clients' outcomes after treatment? "One fairly certain way of ensuring that we ourselves are neither professional placebos nor psychonoxious, is to collect information on outcome for each and every client we see" (Truax & Carkhuff, 1967, p. 369). A routine follow-up call is one possibility. Think how you appreciate it if your doctor calls you after an office visit to see how you're doing. In some contexts, it may even be a reimbursable service, and indeed it can constitute good continuing care. In our own field of addiction treatment, a routine check-in at 3–6 months is an opportunity to catch recurring problems early on and provide further treatment as needed, which is good practice in managing chronic conditions more generally. Beyond the potential benefits to clients, you also gain a bigger picture of the enduring effects of treatment. How might you arrange routine follow-up visits with those under your care?

It is even possible to conduct relatively inexpensive and useful trials within ongoing practice. For example, say you are considering adding a new component to current procedures with the hope that it will improve client outcomes. How would you know whether it does? A fairly simple program evaluation design (Miller, 1980) is to implement the new component on an experimental basis during a trial period, perhaps randomly assigning clients to receive or not receive the additional service (e.g., Bien, Miller, & Boroughs, 1993; J. Brown & Miller, 1993). Alternatively, outcomes of interest might be monitored for a period of time before implementation, then during a trial period of the new procedure, then again returning to standard practice without the innovation (an A-B-A design). If the outcome is one that is easily measured (e.g., the percentage of clients who return for treatment after intake), informative results may be available within a matter of weeks or months.

As mentioned in Chapter 8, a privilege in conducting clinical trials is that we get to learn the outcomes of everyone who was treated, something that doesn't often happen in routine practice. It has given us a clear appreciation of how very well most clients do after treatment (e.g., Anton et al., 2006; Miller, Walters, et al., 2001; Project MATCH Research Group, 1997), in stark contrast to sometimes gloomy public and professional opinion about addiction outcomes based on anecdotes. We also found that most clients appreciate being contacted to learn how they are faring. As an afterthought in a long-term follow-up study, we asked clients to rate the therapist they had seen, and we found that they often named the skillful research assistant who had been conducting their follow-up interviews! As far as they were concerned, it was continuing care.

Research on Deliberate Practice

There is good evidence to support the impact of deliberate practice in achieving skillfulness as a therapist. Daryl Chow and colleagues (2015) used multilevel modeling to examine therapist functioning in a large group of independent practitioners providing services within a practice network. As a part of participating in the network, therapists received feedback about their clients' outcomes at every session through the use of a standardized outcome measure. The study included 69 therapists and their 4,580 clients across 45 different agencies. As usual, some therapists were found to have reliably better outcomes, even when controlling for client severity and therapist training and experience. As others have found (G. S. Brown, Lambert, Jones, & Minami, 2005), there were also therapists who had consistently worse outcomes, even though their clients had about the same level of severity as those seen by the high-performing therapists. There is no getting away from it: Some therapists are just better (or worse) for clients than others. In a subset ($n = 17$) of the most and least effective therapists, those who engaged in more deliberate practice activities were also more likely to be among the high-performing group. In fact, the top-performing therapists spent almost three times as much effort in deliberate practice as the lowest-performing therapists. Chow et al. (2015) also found that *any* of 24 deliberate practice activities were associated with improved client outcomes *in a context where therapists receive regular feedback about client outcomes.* Deliberate practice + feedback = increased expertise and better client outcomes.

Another study supporting the role of deliberate practice in improving clinical expertise followed all therapists and their clients in a large mental health clinic over 7 years. Therapists received routine feedback about client outcomes over this period of time as well as increased consultation when clients were not improving, or the therapist was struggling. A variety of strategies were used to implement deliberate practice for therapists in this agency, including rehearsing difficult conversations, using simulated case vignettes, and reviewing and reflecting on sessions. Over the 7 years in which this quality improvement initiative was implemented, client outcomes steadily improved year by year, both overall and within each therapist's caseload. Note that in this study, deliberate practice was focused on worrisome cases, with active and systematic strategies for doing something different when they were encountered. Thus, it can be valuable to concentrate your deliberate practice on clinical situations where you feel particularly challenged.

Taking charge of your own professional growth is a powerful antidote for the isolation to which our profession is prone. Active engagement in deliberate practice can improve your therapeutic skills, with results reflected in your clients' outcomes.

KEY POINTS

- Practitioners' therapeutic expertise and client outcomes generally do not improve with years of experience.
- Deliberate practice means intentionally engaging in activities designed to improve proficiency through repetition and successive refinement.
- With deliberate practice and feedback, therapeutic expertise and client outcomes can both improve.
- Deliberate practice can be used to improve not only technical, but also interpersonal therapeutic skills that influence client outcomes.

CHAPTER 13

Teaching Therapeutic Skills

At some point in your career, you may find yourself with the responsibility of teaching, supervising, or coaching others. Perhaps this is already an important part of your work. In doing so, you necessarily make choices about what aspects of practice are most important to convey in your teaching, and such decisions mirror larger issues in counseling and psychotherapy. To what extent would you focus on interpersonal skills in your teaching?

Clinical training is often focused on performing specific techniques prescribed within a particular theoretical perspective (Crits-Christoph, Frank, Chambless, Brody, & Karp, 1995). Your trainees might learn how to:

- Teach particular self-regulation skills, distress tolerance, or cognitive restructuring.
- Develop a desensitization hierarchy, clarify personal values, or complete a functional analysis.
- Analyze transference, walk clients through systematic exposure to traumatic events, or repair a rupture in working alliance.

Therapist manuals may be used to improve consistency and fidelity when providing specific treatments (e.g., Barlow, 2014; Carroll, 1998; Linehan, 2014; Martell, Dimidjian, & Herman-Dunn, 2013; Miller, 2004), with adherence being measured by observing and documenting the performance of particular prescribed procedures (Carroll et al., 1998; Miller, Moyers, et al., 2005). Yet, the use of treatment manuals has yielded no consistent improvement in client outcomes (Beidas & Kendall, 2010; Truijens, Zühlke-Van Hulzen, & Vanheule, 2019). Therapist adherence to treatment manuals appears to be insufficient for improving professional expertise and client outcomes.

Although the importance of therapeutic relationship is widely acknowledged, clinical training has not always explored what this means and how it is achieved. In both clinical training and therapist manuals, relatively little attention has often been paid to the therapeutic skills described in this book, even though they appear to impact client outcomes more than do the differences between specific treatment techniques or systems of psychotherapy. In this chapter, we discuss how interpersonal therapist skills can and should be included in clinical teaching, but first we consider three meta-professional roles in the teaching of counselors and psychotherapists: trainer, coach, and supervisor.

Meta-Professional Roles: What Am I Doing Here?

Over the course of a career in delivering individual therapeutic services, you might have a benevolent personal impact in the lives of hundreds of clients. If you have the opportunity to train, supervise, or coach other providers, your influence may be extended to the care of many thousands of people. Teaching expertise is quite a different task from providing therapy, and your own interpersonal skills are vital here as well.

These three meta-professional roles—training, supervising, and coaching—can be confused with each other, in part because they are sometimes blended within service systems. You could be asked to take on more than one of these tasks simultaneously. It's worth considering what you are being asked to do in each of these roles.

Training

We define "training" as the conveying of skills that are needed to improve treatment in some way. This can include:

- Initial clinical training (e.g., graduate education)
- (Re)training in a previously unfamiliar therapeutic skill (e.g., continuing professional education)
- Quality assurance, improving adherence to a treatment method, or recertifying
- Specific content that is important in professional functioning (e.g., ethical guidelines or diagnostic criteria), and
- Ongoing strengthening of interpersonal skills that can improve the quality and outcomes of many different forms of treatment

As we will soon discuss, there is strong evidence that more than didactic instruction is required in order to convey expertise in any of these complex therapeutic skills. This should be no surprise. Imagine providing a classroom workshop on how to play the bassoon, fly an airplane, or remove an inflamed appendix. A lecture can be a good start, but is followed by observed practice and feedback in the context of supervision or coaching. A clear finding in clinical training research is that workshop or classroom instruction alone is unlikely to have much enduring impact on practice (Herschell et al., 2010; *Didactic instruction is* Miller et al., 2006). Nevertheless, *insufficient to convey* a didactic model remains the pre- *expertise in therapeutic skills.* dominant form of continuing professional education in counseling and psychotherapy. In other words, we invest the most time in a type of learning that is least effective for improving clinical skillfulness.

Supervising

"Supervision" is a formal relationship between two providers, one of whom has authority over the other. Supervision extends across time, with the purpose of preventing harm and improving the skills of the supervisee. Supervisors are typically licensed or certified, and are tasked with monitoring the quality of the professional services of supervisees and serving as gatekeepers for a profession (M. V. Ellis et al., 2014; Hill & Knox, 2013). Thus, supervisors are explicitly and often legally accountable for mistakes made by their supervisees. Supervisors have authority to interrupt or redirect the clinical services of supervisees if they see that client care is being compromised.

They can initiate remedial learning plans, and in extreme cases can intervene to prohibit supervisees from providing clinical care entirely. Client safety is a supervisor's first concern and responsibility, with the training needs of supervisees as an important secondary task.

In this kind of relationship, learners may choose to guard carefully what they say and do, because they know that their teacher is evaluating them. This is an unavoidable consequence of the accountability inherent in supervisory roles (Wilson, Davies, & Weatherhead, 2016). As with other clinical activities, supervision should incorporate informed consent, including explicit acknowledgment of the supervisor's authority and responsibilities when concerns are encountered.

Coaching

"Coaching," on the other hand, is a collaborative relationship. Risk management is attended to by a separate supervisor or by the learners themselves, who may be licensed or certified to practice independently. Though the coach presumably has a higher level of expertise, the relationship is not hierarchical, and the consultant has no ability to sanction learners, compel them to remediation, or remove them from practice. Coaches may or may not work within the same organization as the learners, and their role typically does not include explicit organizational accountability for client safety. When coaches know that the safety of clients is being managed elsewhere, they are free to focus on developing their learners' skills.

Coaching goes well beyond providing information. It typically requires directly observing a learner's performance and providing feedback and suggestions for skill improvement. A coaching relationship can extend over time or may be time-limited, as with a visiting consultant or a master class.

Dual roles that blur the tasks of training, supervising, and coaching can be confusing. Think carefully about which teaching role you are taking on in order to avert problems down the line for both yourself and your learners. Do your responsibilities include:

- Conveying information?
- Increasing observable skills, perhaps to a criterion of competence?
- Evaluating knowledge and/or skill acquisition?

- Screening/selecting candidates for training?
- Preventing harm?
- Enhancing motivation to learn in your trainees?

Teaching Therapeutic Skills

We were trained two decades apart at universities with quite different clinical psychology programs. At one, all of the faculty solidly identified as behavior therapists, cautiously skeptical of even cognitive therapy. The other clinical training program was broadly eclectic, with clinicians representing half a dozen divergent and often conflicting schools of psychotherapy. In both training programs, however, the first year-long clinical course, before we ever saw clients, focused on the therapeutic relationship. We learned a facilitative way of working with clients that served as a foundation on which to build other therapeutic skills, as well as a safety net we could always trust to at least do no harm. We think this is a good model in training new counselors and psychotherapists, to first focus on the fundamentals of a therapeutic relationship. A year-long course that specializes in learning these skills is a wise investment for later competence in any psychotherapeutic approach. You can provide beginners with a solid foundation of therapeutic skills that are unlikely to do harm, blend well with and enhance the outcome of other forms of treatment.

The therapeutic skills described in this book can be helpful not only for therapists themselves, but also for others who interact with clients, such as those who answer the telephones, collect information, or schedule appointments (Miller, 2018; Nichols, 2009; Rakel, 2018). Truax and Carkhuff (1967, pp. 107–109) found that after training, there were no significant differences in the therapeutic skill levels of lay counselors, psychology graduate students, and experienced professionals. Our primary focus here, though, is on the preparation of providers of therapeutic services.

Whom to Teach?

How should you decide where to focus your training, supervision, and coaching? It is clear that people vary in their potential ability to develop therapeutic skills. Some seem to have a natural propensity and learn quickly; others may show little progress even with intensive training (Miller et al., 2004; Moyers et al., 2008). There are few guidelines for identifying in advance the candidates who are most likely to have clinical talent. The scientific literature does clarify some factors that *do not* reliably predict the development of therapeutic skills: personality (such as introversion/extroversion), experience, education, gender, and age (Miller et al., 2004). Characteristics and qualifications that appear on a résumé or graduate school application are largely unrelated to the potential effectiveness of a therapist.

So, what *does* indicate learners who are more likely to acquire therapeutic acumen? Some candidates may have a head start in already showing some development of pertinent interpersonal skills. In selecting candidates to learn and provide complex therapies, for example, we found that prescreening for empathic listening skills expedited the learning of motivational interviewing (Miller, Moyers, et al., 2005) and subsequently predicted better client outcomes (Moyers, Houck, et al., 2016). For entry-level training, a probationary period could be used to assess the extent to which candidates show progress in being able to demonstrate therapeutic skills in practice. In scientist–practitioner clinical programs, it might be wise to do this in the first year of training rather than shaping scientific skills only to discover worrisome interpersonal deficits years later. As emphasized in Chapter 2, "Professions should take an active hand in weeding out or retraining therapists, educators, counselors, etc., who are unable to provide high levels of effective ingredients, and who therefore are likely to provide human encounters that change people *for the worse*" (Truax & Carkhuff, 1967, p. 142; italics in original).

Beyond already developed interpersonal skills, a further factor is motivation to learn. Continuing education workshops are quite a different experience depending on whether the learners have chosen and invested personal resources to learn, or have been told, "You're required to learn this whether you like it or not." In introducing new skills in an ongoing system, we have found it far better to begin with those who most want to learn and show best potential, rather than trying to retrain everyone. It is a bit like trying to light many candles with a single match. Preparing a small group of learners to succeed allows them, in turn, to encourage

> *Qualifications on paper are largely unrelated to a therapist's effectiveness.*

others. We believe that choosing a smaller, motivated, and talented group of learners is the best way to implement system change in the long run.

Relevance

A vital foundational message from clinical teachers is that interpersonal skills *matter*. This is not unscientific mumbo jumbo. To the contrary, the impact of interpersonal skills is rooted in the very origins of clinical science in psychology (Miller & Moyers, 2017). Any evidence-based treatment is intertwined with the qualities of those who provide it. Furthermore, a therapeutic skill like accurate empathy *is* an evidence-based component of treatment and has been so for half a century (Elliott et al., 2011b; see Chapter 3).

Attitude

Another foundational perspective in teaching interpersonal therapeutic skills is that they are not merely techniques. Rogers (1980d) emphasized the importance of therapists' underlying "attitude," the mindset or assumptions that guide practice. Therapists in training readily cling to techniques and manuals that can be "the words without the music," conveying a sense of doing something *to* rather than *with* the client (Miller & Rollnick, 2013; Rollnick & Miller, 1995). It matters how you think about your work, how you understand your role.

Ordinarily, attitudes and values are shaped gradually over time through interpersonal interactions, although they can also be transformed by distinct experiences (Ajzen & Fishbein, 1980; Miller & C'de Baca, 1994, 2001; Rokeach, 1973). The teaching of therapeutic attitudes can begin with communicating that they *matter*, encouraging therapist reflection at a deeper level than technique. A "think-aloud" methodology that has been used to study cognition and emotion (Davison, Vogel, & Coffman, 1997) can also be used in clinical training to articulate thoughts that are guiding practice. Either during simulated practice or in reviewing audio- or video-recorded sessions, stop the interaction and ask reflective questions such as:

- "What are (were) you thinking at this point?"
- "Where are you going here?"

- "Why did you ask that particular question?"
- "How are you hoping the client will respond?"
- "Why did you reflect that particular part of what the client said?"

This is not done with a judgmental tone (*"What on earth were you thinking!?"*) but with curiosity to understand and help trainees reflect on how they are processing information.

Demonstration

As mentioned in the Preface, it can be informative to observe the progenitors of particular treatment approaches actually practicing them. To be sure, there will be therapist idiosyncrasies that don't need to be emulated, but the originators of a method may do much that is important and not reflected in their writing or speaking about treatment. It is not just what they do, but *how* they do it. Their interpersonal communications may be at least as important as the specific techniques they describe. In just the same way, it will be important for your students to be able to watch you as you demonstrate how you would approach clinical interactions with a focus on interpersonal skills. How, exactly, might you do things differently if you considered the relationship with the client to be at least as important as the content of the treatment you were delivering? Are you willing to allow your trainees to observe as you interact with clients? In our opinion, an important quality for teachers of counseling and psychotherapy is their willingness to be observed in actual practice.

Observed Practice, Feedback, and Coaching

There is an unspoken and convenient myth that has grown up around observation of practice: that psychotherapy is special magic that can only happen behind closed doors. Of course, there are elements of privacy that make therapy unique, but it is not magic, and observing it does not make it less effective. A clear finding from training research is that therapists benefit from feedback about their work *based on observing their practice*. Such individualized feedback can be partially quantitative as well as qualitative (Beidas & Kendall, 2010;

Miller et al., 2004). Active learning that includes practice and feed-back predicts acquiring and keeping therapy skills, whereas reading or didactic workshop training alone does not (Herschell et al., 2010; Rakovshik, McManus, Vazquez-Montes, Muse, & Ougrin, 2016). Internet protocols can help to strengthen therapeutic skills *if* they include practice and feedback (Kobak, Craske, Rose, & Wolitsky-Taylor, 2013). Another impor-tant reason for observed practice is that therapists are notoriously poor judges of the quality of their own work. The least effective ther-apists rate themselves as being just *Therapists benefit from feedback about their work based on observing their practice.* as competent as the most effective therapists, and dramatically over-estimate their outcomes most of the time (S. D. Miller, Hubble, & Chow, 2017). Despite efforts to increase the economy and scalability of therapist training, there is not yet a viable substitute for expert feedback to learners (Herschell et al., 2010).

Experiential Learning

Engaging trainees in experiential practice is particularly important for developing interpersonal therapeutic skills. Beyond observed practice with clients as described above, it can be useful to struc-ture training exercises to experience and develop these interpersonal skills. Role-play is a common way to do this, in which trainees inter-act with colleagues or actors portraying clients (Ottman, Kohrt, Ped-ersen, & Schafer, 2020). However, even professional actors may not respond as actual clients would, instead portraying a role they have constructed. Clinical trainees or colleagues may portray clients who are too easy on the one hand, or unrealistically intractable and unre-sponsive to interpersonal cues on the other. Taking time to develop a role before beginning can help, as can midpractice adjustments to the role (e.g., in severity or difficulty level). Role-plays also have the advantage of your being able to "rewind" and start again from a particular point while trying a different approach. When we use this option in our training, we ask those who are enacting client roles to respond spontaneously as feels natural within the role, rather than following a preplanned course. Although role-playing with standardized clients can be intimidating for trainees, they usually evaluate it as a valuable part of learning new treatment approaches (Napel-Schutz, Abma, Bamelis, & Arntz, 2017).

A useful alternative to role-play is what we have called "real play," in which interviewees speak about themselves. Such interactions are usually more genuine than enacted roles and facilitate learning for both participants. The interviewer is interacting with a real person who responds naturally. The interviewee, in turn, gets receiving-end experience in responding to therapeutic interpersonal styles. The interviewer is practicing therapeutic skills, and the interviewee is talking about actual experience, though the subject matter need not be deeply therapeutic (Miller, 2018; Nichols, 2009). The interviewer is not trying to fix or change the speaker. It is, in essence, a conversation with a supportive listener.

Of course, both parties in real play are also responding to context: who is observing, the perceived safety of the setting, performance and evaluative anxiety. The interviewee, for example, may choose a seemingly safe topic to begin with, but then the empathic interaction goes farther and deeper than anticipated. Give interviewees explicit permission to exit a real play at any time. A training format we have used to benefit the interviewer instructs all observers to watch for examples of good and skillful practice, and take note of these so that they can be recounted. You can also suggest that interviewers insert an intentional mistake or two!

What to Teach: Practical Components

There is a certain irony to the term "nonspecific," if it is taken to mean that these therapeutic skills cannot be specified or taught. Operationally defining and measuring therapists' interpersonal skills was at the heart of early clinical science, specifying therapeutic processes and linking them to client outcomes (Carkhuff & Truax, 1965; Kirschenbaum, 2009; Miller & Moyers, 2017; Truax & Carkhuff, 1967). Training for these skills was already being developed and evaluated in the 1960s. When operationally defined, the desired skill can be observed and presumably strengthened in practice.

Accurate empathy (Chapter 3) is the most studied of these interpersonal therapeutic skills, and has been found in meta-analyses to bear the strongest relationship to client outcomes (Elliott, Bohart,

Watson, & Greenberg, 2011a; Elliott, Bohart, Watson, &Murphy, 2018). Originally, therapist ratings were made on a Likert scale with narrative descriptions of each level of skill (Truax & Carkhuff, 1967). The practice behavior of reflective listening can be reliably coded and is highly correlated with observers' global ratings of accurate empathy (Villarosa-Hurlocker, O'Sickey, Houck, & Moyers, 2019). Skillfulness in reflective listening can be developed through successive approximations such as nonverbal attending, generating and testing guesses about possible meaning, forming reflective statements, and increasing the ratio of reflections to questions (Egan, 2014; Miller, 2018; Moyers, Martin, Manuel, Hendrickson, & Miller, 2005; Nichols, 2009; Rosengren, 2018).

In addition to improved outcomes, strong interpersonal skills offer therapists another important advantage: the ability to adjust their approach depending on moment-to-moment interactions with their clients. This therapeutic meta-skill of adapting treatments to clients is broadly known as "responsiveness" (Norcross & Wampold, 2019; Stiles, Honos-Webb, & Surko, 1998). Responsive therapists are likely to change what they offer depending on what they encounter with a client, rather than persisting in one approach. Empathy, for example, is a foundational therapeutic skill, but it is also important to observe the client's moment-to-moment responses, and to choose when and how specific skills (including empathy) should be used (Hatcher, 2015). Research indicates that skilled therapists adjust treatment protocols with clients in order to achieve optimal outcomes, despite a researcher's goal of keeping the treatment as uniform as possible (Boswell et al., 2013; Imel, Baer, Martino, Ball, & Carroll, 2011; Zickgraf et al., 2016). This finding is particularly compelling with regard to the level of client resistance (Hatcher, 2015; Karno & Longabaugh, 2005). Competent therapists do not push forward with direction, teaching, or specific protocol tasks when clients are pushing back. Although these studies do not say what therapists do *instead,* it is likely that therapeutic conditions play a critical role. Research is accumulating to indicate that strict adherence to treatment manuals actually compromises client outcomes (A. N. C. Campbell et al., 2015; Miller, Yahne, & Tonigan, 2003; Webb, DeRubeis, & Barber, 2010; Zickgraf et al., 2016), whereas the therapist's ability to respond flexibly to clients after developing competence in a manualized treatment predicts better outcome (Boswell et al., 2013; Elkin et al., 2014; Safran et al., 1990).

In Positions of Influence

Sometimes talented clinicians accept positions in which they can influence the direction of organizational structures through program management and/or policy development. In such positions, clinical science can be applied in continuing quality improvement of client services and professional skills. An administrator who is responsible for hiring new therapists, for example, has an opportunity to foster significant and sometimes rapid change in program atmosphere (Marshall & Nielsen, 2020). When hiring therapists to deliver empirically supported treatments, attending to and prioritizing interpersonal therapeutic skills may improve a program's overall outcomes (Moyers, Houck, et al., 2016; Moyers & Miller, 2013). Training, supervision, and consultation practices can be implemented to strengthen the quality of services within an agency (Rousmaniere, Goodyear, Miller, & Wampold, 2017). Program policies and procedures can be adopted to normalize the observation of service delivery, consistent with the American Psychological Association's requirement of "eyes-on" observation of therapy trainees (American Psychological Association, 2015). Routine measurement of client satisfaction and outcomes can be implemented to further improve services, and may be the only way to detect and respond to outlier providers whose work is well below average or even harmful to clients (Goldberg, Babins-Wagner, & Miller, 2017). Similar quality practices could be encouraged more widely by clinicians who find themselves in leadership positions or on boards of organizations responsible for continuing education, licensing or certification, professional conferences, ethical standards, or the training of new providers.

Professional services have long suffered from a disturbing lag between what is known from science and what is actually implemented in practice (E. M. Rogers, 2003). Much is already known about the efficacy of behavioral health treatment methods. Much is

Routine measurement of client satisfaction and outcomes can improve services.

also known about the qualities of treatment providers that improve or deter client outcomes within evidence-based treatments. This knowledge can be applied in your individual practice, in agency policies that you influence, and in broader professional training and standards when you have a role in developing those. Consider focusing on therapists' interpersonal skills as a way of maximizing your contribution to the improvement of psychotherapy, particularly as your influence widens beyond the therapy room.

KEY POINTS

- The teaching of evidence-based therapeutic interpersonal skills should begin early in the training of counselors and psychotherapists.

- The meta-professional roles of training, supervising, and coaching have different functions in teaching new and continuing treatment providers.

- There have been few reliable guidelines for identifying in advance the candidates who are most likely to have clinical talent.

- It is important for teachers to profess and model that therapeutic interpersonal skills matter and are evidence-based.

- These therapeutic skills are not merely techniques, but reflect and express an underlying attitude or mindset.

- An important quality for teachers of counseling and psychotherapy is willingness to be observed in actual practice.

CHAPTER 14

Toward a Broader Clinical Science

When Carl Rogers became its president in 1947, the American Psychological Association was a consortium of experimental specialties that included few clinicians and largely shunned or at least ignored counseling and psychotherapy as unscientific (Kirschenbaum, 2009). Rogers's commitment to clinical science was arguably his most important professional contribution to psychology. Like the reflections that he offered to clients, he regarded his broader ideas not as settled fact but as approximations and hypotheses to be tested (Miller & Moyers, 2017).

Conceptions of clinical science have both sharpened and narrowed since Rogers's seminal work. We have at our disposal far better measures for evaluating treatment efficacy. In clinical trials through the 1960s, the impact of clinical interventions was often assessed by relatively crude measures such as the Minnesota Multiphasic Personality Inventory (MMPI) scale scores (e.g., Rogers et al., 1967). Furthermore, it no longer suffices, at least in scientific journals, simply to say that one delivered a brand-name therapy. It is now expected in clinical science, if not in practice, that there be some measure of treatment fidelity beyond therapist self-report of what was actually delivered. In turn, the observer ratings often used for fidelity monitoring have facilitated the exploration of underlying therapeutic mechanisms, with the unsettling finding that psychotherapies often do not work for the predicted reasons (e.g., Longabaugh

& Wirtz, 2001). The specification and testing of explanatory causal chains is a demanding standard in clinical research and is precisely what Rogers and his students pioneered, with direct implications for what to focus on in clinical training (Kirschenbaum, 2009; Truax & Carkhuff, 1967, 1976). When hypothesized therapeutic mechanisms are identified and operationally defined, they can be experimentally tested (e.g., Glynn & Moyers, 2010; Longabaugh & Wirtz, 2001; Nock, 2007; Magill et al., 2015; Truax & Carkhuff, 1965). A full causal chain would demonstrate that clinical training changes practice behaviors that, in turn, impact therapeutic processes to demonstrably improve treatment outcome (M. Magill & Hallgren, 2019; Moyers et al., 2009).

At the same time, relative to the work of Rogers, current clinical science has had a somewhat narrowed vision focusing on the efficacy of specific treatment techniques. One result of this focus has been the development of lists of "evidence-based" treatments, with encouragement to train and reimburse only those procedures on the list, paralleling the billing codes used in medical care. What appears on such lists, of course, depends on the rules of evidence and burden of proof: How much of what kind(s) of scientific findings suffice to designate a brand-name treatment as "effective"? A National Registry of Evidence-Based Programs and Practices (NREPP) set the evidential bar so low as to generate a list of 479 effective interventions (Gorman, 2017). Shorter diagnosis-specific lists vary in content depending on how evidence is weighed (e.g., Chambless et al., 1998; Miller & Wilbourne, 2002).

Specific Treatments or Therapeutic Relationship?

A polarized debate emerged between proponents of specific evidence-based treatment procedures and advocates of the importance of therapeutic relationship, though there have been some signs of integration (Hofmann & Barlow, 2014). Is what matters in therapy the specific procedures being used or the relational context within which they are delivered? The problem with this question is the word "or." Clearly, both matter, and an either/or dichotomy is misleading (Miller & Moyers, 2015). Few would argue that it makes no difference what a counselor does. Yet, it is also true that when different *bona fide* behavioral treatment procedures are compared in randomized clinical trials, their average outcomes are usually similar. Even unspecified "treatment as usual" may produce outcomes comparable to those from highly structured, manual-guided and closely supervised psychotherapies (Wells, Saxon, Calsyn, Jackson, & Donovan, 2010; Westerberg, Miller, & Tonigan, 2000). Furthermore, specific treatment procedures are inseparable from the people who provide them (Okamoto, Dattilio, Dobson, & Kazantzis, 2019). Even when strong efforts are made to standardize treatment delivery, clients' outcomes still vary with the therapists who treated them (Crits-Christoph, Baranackie, Kurcias, & Beck, 1991; Kim et al., 2006; Miller & Moyers, 2015; Mulder, Murray, & Rucklidge, 2017; Project MATCH Research Group, 1998).

> *Specific treatment procedures are inseparable from the people who provide them.*

Implementation

There are further complexities in the dissemination, implementation, and quality control of treatment methods. Clinical trials of psychotherapies are usually conducted under highly controlled conditions, and a treatment's effect size tends to shrink when it is subsequently implemented in community practice (Miller et al., 2006). Ironically, although treatments themselves may be evidence-based, there is often very little scientific basis for the methods that are used to train, disseminate, and implement them (Fixsen et al., 2005, 2019; McHugh & Barlow, 2010). Thus, what is actually delivered in community practice can be quite different from the specific treatment procedures originally tested. Without close auditing of actual practice, a requirement to deliver evidence-based treatment reduces to little more than claiming to do so (Miller & Meyers, 1995).

Treatment Manuals

One strategy for improving treatment fidelity has been the publication of detailed procedure manuals for therapists to follow. In order to obtain funding for clinical trials of behavioral interventions, researchers must specify the treatment procedures to be tested. This is a reasonable requirement, and treatment manuals thus emerged as a by-product of clinical trials in which the delivery of treatment is usually closely monitored and supervised. For quality assurance, therapists who drift from the specified procedures during a clinical trial may be "red-lined," preventing them from treating any further cases until their adherence improves (e.g., Miller, Moyers, et al., 2005). Therapist manuals are then disseminated for use in community practice, often with little or no special training, monitoring, or quality control. Even within clinical trials, there is little evidence that following a detailed manual significantly improves treatment outcome (Truijens et al., 2019). In a meta-analysis (Hettema et al., 2005) of clinical trials of motivational interviewing, for example, the average effect size was substantially larger in studies that did *not* use a manual for standardization ($d = 0.65 \pm 0.62$) than in studies where treatment was manual-guided ($d = 0.37 \pm 0.62$). Other meta-analyses have found small effects favoring trials with manuals (Crits-Christoph et al., 1991), but direct within-study randomized comparisons have shown no difference in outcomes of manual-guided versus non-manual-guided therapist delivery (Ghaderi, 2006) or client self-directed change (Miller & Baca, 1983; Miller et al., 1980; van Oppen et al., 2010). One large study determined that higher therapist adherence to a manual was associated with lower client retention (B. K. Campbell, Guydish, Le, Wells, & McCarty, 2015). In community practice, average outcomes of manual-guided treatments have been found to be no different from those of unstandardized treatment as usual (e.g., Wells et al., 2010; Westerberg et al., 2000).

> *There is little evidence that following a detailed manual significantly improves treatment outcome.*

Toward Integration in Clinical Science

In recent decades, clinical research has devoted far more attention to the testing of specific treatment procedures than to the impact of how they are actually delivered and the people who provide them (Laska, Gurman, & Wampold, 2014). Though omnipresent, therapist effects are often regarded as nuisance variance to be minimized. Yet, specific psychotherapies are delivered by providers who influence outcomes (Kim et al., 2006; Luborsky et al., 1997; Okiishi et al., 2003; Wampold & Bolt, 2006). The same may be true for pharmaco-therapies, and here even less attention has been given to the provider–patient relationship. In multisite trials, treatment effects are averaged across sites, often regarding as irrelevant the fact that the medication or psychotherapy "works" at some sites and not others (Anton et al., 2006; Ball et al., 2007).

William Miller and Gary Rose (2009, 2010) suggested differen-tiating "technical" (specific procedures) and "relational" components of a behavioral intervention. Yet, even a technical/relational dichot-omy is somewhat arbitrary because relational components such as accurate empathy, acceptance, and affirmation are still expressed and studied as therapist behavior. This does not mean that rela-tional factors are *nothing more* than therapist responses, but it is through counselors' observable behavior that relational components are conveyed to clients and accessible to clinical science. Referring to relational components as "nonspecific" is unhelpful. If they are learnable, measurable, and matter in treatment outcome, then they should be specified, studied, and included in clinical research and training. That is what was happening in the beginnings of clinical sci-ence: seeking to define, study, and teach relational components that matter in treatment (Truax & Carkhuff, 1967, 1976). Rogers (1957) described core relational conditions as "necessary and sufficient." We concur with Rogers that these are necessarily components of effective clinical practice and training, though not always sufficient in them-selves (Hofmann & Barlow, 2014). To assert that a good therapeutic relationship is *sufficient* is to imply that nothing else matters in treat-ment, an absurd claim in health care more generally. It would assert that we have no active psychological treatments except for therapeu-tic relationship.

It is reasonable to ask whether a particular treatment exerts a specific benefit beyond the salutary effects of relational factors (e.g., Singla et al., 2020). This is psychotherapy's closest parallel to a placebo control condition in pharmacotherapy research. There is no direct parallel to placebo when clinicians know what treatment they are delivering and have expectations about it—a problem when-ever therapists and treatment conditions are "crossed" (i.e., two or more treatments delivered by the same providers). In this kind of crossed design, the added potential exists for contamination between treatment conditions (N. Magill, Knight, McCrone, Ismail, & Landau, 2019). In "nested" designs (when two or more treatments are delivered by different providers who have confidence in the approach that they are using), designating one of the treatments to be a placebo simply means that the investigator does not believe in its efficacy. Investigator allegiance effects (i.e., the investigator's favorite treatment "wins") do occur, but not always. In Project MATCH (1997), for example, site differences indicated that, if anything, the principal investigator's cherished treatment fared worse than the competition.

Provider and treatment cannot be unconfounded, but both technical and relational components can be measured and studied as potentially active ingredients in order to understand better what is happening in counseling and psychotherapy. Both technical and relational aspects of treatment can contribute to positive outcomes (Hofmann & Barlow, 2014; Schwartz, Chambless, McCarthy, Milrod, & Barber, 2019), and there is no particular reason to assume that one depends entirely on the other. For example, in a complex, manual-guided, cognitive-behavioral therapy for alcohol misuse, both

> *Both technical and relational components can be measured and studied as potentially active ingredients.*

specific content (e.g., strategies for managing cravings) and relational attributes (therapist empathy) made independent contributions to client outcome (Moyers, Houck, et al., 2016).

In this section, we consider four interrelated elements of behavioral science that apply equally to technical and relational components of counseling and psychotherapy: (1) definition and measurement of key variables, (2) practice–process linkage, (3) process–outcome linkage, and (4) training–practice linkage. We will illustrate each of these linkages from recent research on motivational interviewing.

Definition and Measurement of Key Variables

Careful observation is the beginning of science. Which client outcomes matter, and how can they be operationally defined and measured? Clinical trials customarily specify a target outcome as the primary dependent measure at a particular endpoint. Program evaluation in community treatment similarly specifies and measures the intended outcomes of delivered services.

What measurable processes are hypothesized to be important in effecting these outcomes? This is the domain of treatment "mechanism" research, and can include measures of both therapist and client in-session responses. Measures of therapist competence have often focused on treatment fidelity, on adhering to prescribed (and sometimes manual-guided) responses. Fidelity checklists of clinical procedures may be completed by therapist self-report or by session observers: Were particular procedures (such as assessing high-risk situations) delivered and, if so, how well (e.g., Carroll et al., 1998)? Observers can also perform ratings on global measures such as therapist empathy that are arrayed on a Likert scale. Global ratings can be combined with specific therapist and client behavior counts (e.g., the number of affirmations a therapist offered) to study treatment processes (e.g., Chamberlain, Patterson, Reid, Kavanagh, & Forgatch, 1984; Miller & Mount, 2001; Moyers, Rowell, et al., 2016; Patterson & Forgatch, 1985). Both technical and relational components of treatment can and should be assessed.

Key Variables: Illustration from Motivational Interviewing Research

In early studies of motivational interviewing (MI), we had the benefit of working in the treatment of alcohol use disorders, a field with already well-developed outcome measures, with a primary focus on the reduction of alcohol consumption and related problems (Litten & Allen, 1992; Miller, Tonigan, & Longabaugh, 1995). It remained to hypothesize what MI-related processes would be important to measure. Because therapist self-report tends to be, at best, modestly related to observer and client ratings of what actually occurred in treatment sessions, we developed a detailed observation system termed the MI Skill Code (MISC; DeJonge, Schippers, & Schaap, 2005; Miller & Mount, 2001; Moyers, Martin, Catley, Harris, & Ahluwalia, 2003). The original MISC was overinclusive, requiring hours of work to code a 20-minute treatment segment reliably. It included mutually exclusive codes for both therapist and client responses (allowing for treatment process coding), global ratings, and recording of relative talk time of client and therapist. A reduced MI Treatment Integrity (MITI) code subsequently focused only on therapist responses and was refined through several revisions to improve reliability and remove redundant or irrelevant codes (Moyers, Rowell, et al., 2016;

Pierson et al., 2007). The MITI, and other scales that measure the quality of delivered treatment, can serve a dual purpose in that they may also inform therapists about how to improve their own practice.

Practice–Process Linkage

Here, observation is focused on relationships between therapist and client responses during treatment. How do prescribed (and proscribed) therapist practices impact relevant in-session treatment processes? What changes in client behavior are influenced by the therapist, and how? What practice behaviors of what quality by which providers produce particular in-session events for which clients? Compared to process–outcome linkage, these relationships may be easier to detect because client and counselor responses occur close in time (within seconds of each other) and are similarly measured by observer coding (M. Magill & Hallgren, 2019).

Predicted practice–process linkages and intervention procedures may be derived from preexisting or emergent theory (S. C. Hayes, 2004; Miller, Toscova, Miller, & Sanchez, 2000; Moos, 2007). The fact that a treatment arose from a particular theory, however, does not mean that it necessarily works for theory-based reasons (e.g., Morgenstern & Longabaugh, 2000). For cognitive-behavioral treatments, an improvement in client skills is a logical explanation for why the treatment works. Yet at least in treating alcohol use disorders, multiple studies have demonstrated that the effect of cognitive-behavioral therapies does not depend on client skill gains (Longabaugh & Magill, 2011; Morgenstern & Longabaugh, 2000). Others have found that skill increases were linked to improvement but occurred equally in cognitive-behavioral and other kinds of treatment (Kadden, Litt, & Cooney, 1992). It is clear that much more careful research is needed to support even simple claims of name-brand treatments concerning practice–process links (M. Magill, Kiluk, McCrady, Tonigan, & Longabaugh, 2015).

The fact that a treatment arose from a particular theory does not mean it works for theory-based reasons.

Hypothesized practice–process relationships can be examined between preselected therapist and client responses. In behavioral analysis, for example, particular client in-session responses can be influenced by positive and negative reinforcement of clinically relevant behaviors (R. J. Kohlenberg & Tsai, 2007; C. K. Shaw & Shrum, 1972). In person-centered counseling, "experiencing" is a clinically relevant client response (Gendlin, 1961; Kiesler, 1971; M. H. Klein et al., 1986) that can be both positively and negatively influenced by counselor practice behavior (Hill et al., 1988; Wiser & Goldfried, 1998).

It is also possible to examine actual practice–process relationships during sessions in order to discover linkages (Varble, 1968). This still involves choosing the client and counselor responses to be observed, although new categories of response or unexpected linkages may emerge during observation. In this regard, it can be beneficial to bring a beginner's mind to the study of clinical practice. Neither client-centered counseling nor MI began with a theory (Kirschenbaum, 2009; Miller & Moyers, 2017). Both arose from observation of practice to develop testable hypotheses about what actually improves client outcomes, with theory emerging later (Miller & Rose, 2009; Rogers, 1959). Of course, the training and experience of progenitors do inform their hypotheses and what client and therapist responses they choose to observe.

Practice–Process Linkage: Illustration from Motivational Interviewing Research

In the earliest formulations of MI, "self-motivational statements" were described as a key clinically relevant behavior (Miller, 1983; Miller & Rollnick, 1991). Later termed "change talk," these are client verbalizations that bespeak movement toward a specific target change. If smoking cessation is the goal of consultation, for example, then "I think I need to quit smoking" is change talk, whereas "I need to quit drinking" is not (though it would be if alcohol cessation were a goal). Psycholinguist Paul Amrhein helped us understand change talk as a category that includes different speech acts signaling desire (I want to), ability (I could), reasons (If . . . then), need (I have to), and commitment (I will) (Amrhein et al., 2003; Miller & Rollnick, 2013). As discussed in Chapter 9, similar verbalizations can be made on behalf of the status quo and were termed "sustain talk." In early research, we unfortunately lumped sustain talk into a broader category of "resistance," but now recognize that sustain talk is merely one side of clients' normal ambivalence. An observational measure of ambivalence is the person's "decisional balance" of change talk and sustain talk.

The relevance of change and sustain talk to client outcomes will be discussed in the next section. For practice–process linkage, it was important to demonstrate that counselor behavior can influence clients' verbalized decisional balance (Miller & Rose, 2009, 2015; Moyers et al., 2017). This linkage has been supported by several types of research. Conditional probabilities from sequential analysis of in-session responses showed that MI-consistent practice behaviors increased the likelihood the client's next utterance would be change talk, whereas MI-inconsistent responses were more likely to be followed by sustain talk (Moyers & Martin, 2006). In another study (Villarosa-Hurlocker et al., 2019), therapist relational skills (empathy, acceptance, collaboration, and autonomy support) had no direct effect on client change talk (cf., M. Magill et al., 2019); rather, providers with high relational skills were more likely to also use the technical skills (such as specific reflection of change talk) to strengthen client change language. It was technical skill *in the context of* relational skill.

Simple correlations of practice behavior with client processes are inconclusive in themselves. It could be, for example, that clients who express plentiful change talk are more likely to evoke empathy and reflections from their counselors. This is why it is important to keep the *order* of the therapist–client interactions intact when examining simple associations. By keeping track of what clients say immediately after therapists offer, for example, an empathic reflection, one can measure whether change talk will decrease or increase. Doing that over the course of an entire session, one can generate conditional probabilities in the form of if-then statements: If the therapist offers an empathic reflection, then the chance of change talk increases. It is the linking of therapist and client statements to each other in time that allows a stronger causal inference (Moyers et al., 2009; Nock, 2007).

Experimental manipulation of practice behavior offers a still stronger line of evidence. In an early study, clients were randomly assigned in a crossed design to therapists who were either more directive and confrontive when encountering resistance, or who responded in a more MI-consistent way (Miller et al., 1993). Clients in the

MI-consistent condition emitted 3.4 times more change talk than resistance, as compared with equal amounts of both (i.e., ambivalence) in the more confrontive condition. Within-subject experiments have yielded similar findings. When family therapists alternated in 12-minute segments between a directive teaching style and an empathic listening style, client resistance increased and decreased (respectively) in step function (Patterson & Forgatch, 1985). In a similar experimental design (Glynn & Moyers, 2010), therapists alternated 12-minute segments of MI or functional analysis. Clients' ratio of change talk to sustain talk averaged 1.8 with MI and 1.0 (ambivalence) with functional analysis.

Process–Outcome Linkage

Does all of this matter? It may be intellectually interesting but clinically irrelevant if the processes being influenced by practice are unrelated to client outcomes. In process–outcome research, the focus is on what are clinically relevant behaviors, processes that can be observed during treatment that are linked to better outcome (R. J. Kohlenberg & Tsai, 2007). What in-session events predict what outcomes of what treatment for what problems at what point in time?

Linking particular processes to successful change is not a new concept. It has been a primary focus within the transtheoretical approach (Prochaska, 1994; Prochaska & DiClemente, 1984; Prochaska & Velicer, 1997) and has been a basis of searching for general evidence-based principles or processes rather than specific treatment procedures (Anthony, 2003; Anthony & Mizock, 2014; Battersby et al., 2010). Behavioral interventions can involve a wide range of processes, some of which may be specific to the intervention, whereas others are more general factors. The transtheoretical model has generated a set of 10 common processes that underlie both therapist-guided and self-directed change (Prochaska & Velicer, 1997).

Large randomized clinical trials (RCTs) powered to detect small treatment effects are not the only, nor even necessarily the best, methodology for discovering process–outcome linkages. If a change principle or process is robust, it should be observable in small trials, quasi-experiments, and even single-subject designs (Ferster & Skinner, 1957). RCTs of specific treatment procedures or program structures tend to be highly expensive and inefficient, and skip an important step by trying to link practice directly to outcome. They typically presume that it is the programmatic structure of different treatments that is important, "when in fact the programs may have been very similar (positively, negatively, or both) in what really matters—that is, the process occurring between service recipients and practitioners" (Anthony, 2003, p. 7).

If a change principle or process is robust, it should be observable in small trials.

It would seem that establishing the nature and strength of process–outcome links is a prerequisite to testing treatment practices to influence the clinically relevant processes. The testing of hypothesized causal mechanisms that underlie treatment effects has been a relatively recent and by no means universal emphasis in clinical outcome research. Yet, it is not new. The work of Charles Truax and Robert Carkhuff (1967) focused on demonstrating both practice–process and process–outcome linkages. Client experiencing, for example, predicts symptomatic improvement (Pascuel-Leone & Yervomenko, 2017). Trials that merely test specific treatment practices in relation to client outcomes skip an intermediate step. As previously discussed, studies explicitly testing this intermediate step have often found that evidence-based treatments do not work for the hypothesized reasons (Longabaugh, Magill, Morgenstern, & Huebner, 2013; Longabaugh & Wirtz, 2001).

We do not mean to privilege either relational or technical aspects of treatment, which at least within talk therapies are functionally intertwined. Both are testable contributors to treatment outcome (Norcross & Wampold, 2011). The relative importance of technical and relational elements may vary by the allegedly specific treatment being studied, by client or cultural factors (Sue & Sue, 2015), or by the condition being addressed (Hofmann & Barlow, 2014). It appears, for example, that the therapeutic relationship may be particularly important in treating addictions (Miller et al., 2019; Najavits & Weiss, 1994). It is conceivable that relational factors may contribute less when a specific treatment is highly effective (e.g., with antibiotic medication). Yet, the opposite is also possible. When an effective intervention is difficult to tolerate, or retention and adherence are vital over an extended period of time, the quality of therapeutic relationship may be crucial. In a meta-analysis (Hettema et al., 2005), when MI (a relational, client-centered method) was combined with other established treatments, the beneficial effect on client outcome was more sustained across 12 months of follow-up.

Process–Outcome Linkage: Illustration from Motivational Interviewing Research

A prediction in early formulations of MI was that client change talk would be linked to subsequent behavior change. Although this linkage has been observed in various studies (Bertholet et al., 2010; T. Martin, Christopher, Houck, & Moyers, 2011; Moyers, Martin, Christopher, et al., 2007; Moyers, Martin, Houck, et al., 2009; Vader et al., 2010), an unexpected finding has been that client sustain talk is often a stronger (and inverse) predictor of outcome (Baer et al., 2008; S. D. Campbell et al., 2010; M. Magill, Apodaca, et al., 2018; M. Magill, Gaume, et al., 2014). That is, outcomes are more strongly (and negatively) predicted by clients' arguments against change than by their arguments for change. What may be even more important, then, is counseling in a way that minimizes client sustain talk, which tends to be evoked and strengthened by MI-inconsistent practice (M. Magill, Gaume, et al., 2014; Miller et al., 1993). Both change talk and sustain talk can be taken into account as predictors by measuring the ratio between them (Moyers, Houck, et al., 2016; Moyers, Martin, et al., 2009). In research with multiple dependent variables, change talk may predict some outcome measures, while sustain talk predicts others (e.g., Marker, Salvaris, Thompson, Tolliday, & Norton, 2019).

The direct impact of relational ("MI spirit") measures tends to be modest (McCambridge, Day, Thomas, & Strang, 2011). However, relational factors can mediate or moderate the impact of technical skills in MI (M. Magill et al., 2018). In one study, low-frequency theoretically MI-inconsistent therapist responses (such as warning, directing, or confronting) *positively* influenced client outcomes, but only when done in the context of strong clinician interpersonal skills such as empathy, acceptance, and genuineness (Moyers, Miller, et al., 2005). Donald Forrester and colleagues (2019) used observational coding of social worker child-in-need visits with families. The worker's interpersonal skills (e.g., empathy) predicted immediate and 20-week family engagement, but not family outcomes, which instead were strongly predicted by the worker's technical skill of evocation.

Training–Practice Linkage

Thus far in this chapter, we have considered practice–process and process–outcome linkages. A remaining testable link is between training and practice. If there are particular technical or relational processes that define a treatment approach (and, ideally, influence client outcomes), then clinical training should demonstrably affect those processes in practice behavior. What training procedures of what duration produce which changes in practice behaviors of what providers? This depends on knowing what practice behaviors are most important, and practice behaviors are necessarily embedded in relational and contextual frames.

Competence and adherence in delivering specific treatment procedures can be measured by observational practice behavior checklists (e.g., Godley et al., 2001; Nuro et al., 2005) or rating scales (e.g., Hill, O'Grady, & Elkin, 1992; Vallis, Shaw, & Dobson, 1986). Relational processes, in contrast, are usually measured via global rating scales rather than specific behavior counts (Colosimo & Pos, 2015; McLeod & Weisz, 2005; Moyers, Rowell, et al., 2016; Truax & Carkhuff, 1976). Observational coding systems can include both technical and relational components of practice (Hill et al., 1992; Moyers, Rowell, et al., 2016).

When evaluated at all, the outcomes of clinical training have most often been documented within clinical trials to establish the delivered fidelity of specific interventions. Less research has focused on the efficacy of clinical training in academic and professional degree programs, or on the impact of continuing professional education. Nevertheless, it is a common finding that changes in practice behavior are minimal and poorly maintained with classroom or workshop training alone (e.g., Miller et al., 2006). This should be unsurprising, in that informational training alone is rarely sufficient to develop proficiency in complex skills.

Training–Practice Linkage: Illustration from Motivational Interviewing Research

Research on MI training began with a shock. Counselors ($n = 22$) participating in a 2-day clinical workshop with the original developer of MI (WRM) provided samples of sessions with actual clients both before and after training (Miller & Mount, 2001). A posttraining practice sample was also obtained with simulated-client actors. In contrast to glowing self-reports of gains in MI skill, observed practice behavior changed modestly at best and quickly returned toward baseline. Unaffected was the frequency of MI-inconsistent counseling responses, which as discussed above may be detrimental to client outcome. Furthermore, client in-session responses (a proxy of subsequent behavioral outcome) changed not at all. Finally, counselors reported being significantly *less* interested in learning more about MI after training than they had been at the outset, a finding that they explained as "we already learned it."

> *Changes in practice behavior are minimal and poorly maintained with classroom or workshop training alone.*

This humbling study raised the better question: "What *does* it take to help counselors develop skillfulness in MI?" We subsequently found in a randomized trial of training methods that individual feedback and coaching—two common aids in learning any complex skill—yielded significant improvement in MI skills that maintained across 12 months (Miller et al., 2004). When examining client in-session responses, only trainees who had received both feedback and coaching after initial training were successful in significantly increasing client change talk.

Another training experiment (Moyers et al., 2017) evaluated MI workshops as usual with a condition-intensifying instruction in the technical component of evoking change talk. We hypothesized that enhancing this language focus for therapists would impact both change talk and sustain talk more than for therapists who did not get this special focus. This was an indirect way of experimentally manipulating one of the treatment elements in MI: how much attention the therapist places on evoking change talk and softening sustain talk. As hypothesized, therapists in the enhanced language training showed reductions in the amount of sustain talk from their clients compared to those trained without the enhanced language focus. There was no differential impact on client change talk, however, which may be related to the fact that a large percentage of clients enrolled in the study had been mandated to treatment—a population for whom softening sustain talk is of prime importance.

In sum, it is possible through clinical training to improve MI practice behaviors that significantly influence client outcomes. MI research to date has supported all three causal links: training to practice, practice to process, and process to outcome.

Integrative Training

Clinical training in both behavioral health and medicine is meant to shape practice behavior, thereby improving treatment outcomes and preventing harm. Yet, research on counseling and psychotherapy training points to modest (at best) gains in trainees' ability to demonstrate competence in delivering evidence-based treatments. A further question is the extent to which learned skills will persist in subsequent practice (Hall, Staiger, Simpson, Best, & Lubman, 2016).

In what technical and relational skills should behavioral health professionals develop (and be able to demonstrate) competence? Theoretical orientations vary in practice behaviors that are prescribed and proscribed. Fidelity to technical procedures of a specific treatment can be assessed, as is now commonly expected in clinical trials (Henggeler, Melton, Brondino, Scherer, & Hanley, 1997; Miller & Rollnick, 2014). Quality of relational aspects of practice can also be reliably measured (Moyers, Houck, et al., 2016; Norcross, 2011; Truax & Carkhuff, 1976).

Logically, clinical training should focus on preparing professionals to deliver treatment that will impact important client processes that facilitate benevolent outcomes. At least as important ethically is to help providers "first, do no harm," to avoid or change any practices that are likely to provoke resistance and adverse outcomes. Truax and Carkhuff (1967) were optimistic in asserting,

> ""We are approaching the point in the development of our field where we will no longer tolerate—even in ourselves, much less in clinics, hospitals and agencies—a failure to keep objective and adequate detailed records of each therapist's effects on patients. We are approaching the point where the laissez-faire attitude that allows many nontherapeutic practices under the name of therapy will no longer be tolerated" (p. 377).

Strengthening Community Practice

Ultimately, the hope of clinical science is to improve the quality and outcomes of prevention and treatment services delivered in routine health care. Clinical trials alone affect few participants unless their lessons are disseminated to and implemented in community practice.

Although relational elements such as accurate empathy have

been described as "common factors," it is unclear just how common they are in practice. Certainly, they are not universal, and providers vary widely in their expression. Acknowledging the importance of therapeutic relationship has implications not only for research, but also for clinical selection, hiring, training, and quality assurance.

One of our intentions is for this volume to serve as a call for greater attention to therapeutic relationship in clinical practice, research, and training. Clinical science began with therapeutic relationship, but of late has focused almost exclusively on technical procedures and mechanisms. Such technique is inseparable from the human beings who provide treatment, and who, we hope, understand themselves as far more than technicians. A clinical science that recognizes the value of both technical and relational components will go a long way to further improve the quality of health care. Renewed focus on therapeutic relationship may also afford greater meaning and joy in the practice of counseling and psychotherapy, further humanizing the services that we provide.

KEY POINTS

- From its original attention to therapeutic processes, clinical science has narrowed to focus on the efficacy of specific treatment techniques.

- Both technical and relational aspects of treatment matter, and are measurable and learnable.

- Particular attention to practice behaviors that compromise client improvement or cause harm is warranted.

- Research in counseling and psychotherapy should define and measure key variables, linking practice behavior to process variables, and processes to outcome.

- Clinical training should be evaluated to show that it affects practice behaviors relevant to therapeutic processes and outcomes.

- Ultimately, the hope of clinical science is to improve the quality of prevention and treatment services delivered in routine care.

References

Ackerman, S. J., & Hilsenroth, M. J. (2003). A review of therapist characteristics and techniques positively impacting the therapeutic alliance. *Clinical Psychology Review, 23*(1), 1–33.

Ajzen, I., & Fishbein, N. (1980). *Understanding attitudes and predicting social behavior*. Englewood Cliffs, NJ: Prentice-Hall.

American Psychiatric Association. (1980). *Diagnostic and statistical manual of mental disorders* (3rd ed.). Washington, DC: Author.

American Psychological Association. (2015). Guidelines for clinical supervision in health service psychology. *American Psychologist, 70*(1), 33–46.

Amrhein, P. C., Miller, W. R., Yahne, C., Knupsky, A., & Hochstein, D. (2004). Strength of client commitment language improves with therapist training in motivational interviewing. *Alcoholism-Clinical and Experimental Research, 28*(5), 74A.

Amrhein, P. C., Miller, W. R., Yahne, C. E., Palmer, M., & Fulcher, L. (2003). Client commitment language during motivational interviewing predicts drug use outcomes. *Journal of Consulting and Clinical Psychology, 71*, 862–878.

Anderson, S. C. (1968). Effects of confrontation by high- and low-functioning therapists. *Journal of Counseling Psychology, 15*(5), 411–416.

Anderson, T., Crowley, M. E. J., Himawan, L., Holmberg, J. K., & Uhlin, D. (2016). Therapist facilitative interpersonal skills and training status: A randomized clinical trial on alliance and outcome. *Psychotherapy Research, 26*(5), 511–529.

Anderson, T., McClintock, A. S., Himawan, L., Song, X., & Patterson, C. L. (2016). A prospective study of therapist facilitative interpersonal skills as a predictor of treatment outcome. *Journal of Consulting and Clinical Psychology, 84*, 57–66.

Anderson, T., Ogles, B. M., Patterson, C. L., Lambert, M. J., & Vermeersch, D. A. (2009). Therapist effects: Facilitative interpersonal skills as a predictor of therapist success. *Journal of Clinical Psychology, 65*(7), 755–768.

Anonymous. (1957). *The cloud of unknowing* (I. Progoff, Trans.). New York: Delta Books.

Anthony, W. A. (2003). Studying evidence-based processes, not practices. *Psychiatric Services, 54*(1), 7.

Anthony, W. A., & Mizock, L. (2014). Evidence-based processes in an era of recovery: Implications for rehabilitation counseling and research. *Rehabilitation Counseling Bulletin, 57*(4), 219–227.

Anton, R. F., O'Malley, S. S., Ciraulo, D. A., Cisler, R. A., Couper, D., Donovan, D. M., . . . Zweben, A. (2006). Combined pharmacotherapies and behavioral interventions for alcohol dependence. *Journal of the American Medical Association, 295*(17), 2003.

Apodaca, T. R., Jackson, K. M., Borsari, B., Magill, M., Longabaugh, R., Mastroleo, N. R., & Barnett, N. P. (2016). Which individual therapist behaviors elicit client change talk and sustain talk in motivational interviewing? *Journal of Substance Abuse Treatment, 61*, 60–65.

Armstrong, K. (2010). *Twelve steps to a compassionate life.* New York: Knopf.

Aveyard, P., Begh, R., Parsons, A., & West, R. (2012). Brief opportunistic smoking cessation interventions: A systematic review and meta-analysis to compare advice to quit and offer of assistance. *Addiction, 107*(6), 1066–1073.

Azrin, N. H. (1976). Improvements in the community-reinforcement approach to alcoholism. *Behaviour Research and Therapy, 14*, 339–348.

Azrin, N. H., Sisson, R. W., Meyers, R. J., & Godley, M. (1982). Alcoholism treatment by disulfiram and community reinforcement therapy. *Journal of Behavior Therapy and Experimental Psychiatry, 13*, 105–112.

Babor, T. F. (2004). Brief treatments for cannabis dependence: Findings from a randomized multisite trial. *Journal of Consulting and Clinical Psychology, 72*, 455–466.

Baer, J. S., Beadnell, B., Garrett, J. A., Hartzler, B., Wells, E. A., & Peterson, P. L. (2008). Adolescent change language within a brief motivational intervention and substance use outcomes. *Psychology of Addictive Behaviors, 22*, 570–575.

Baldwin, S. A., Wampold, B. E., & Imel, Z. E. (2007). Untangling the alliance-outcome correlation: Exploring the relative importance of therapist and patient variability in the alliance. *Journal of Consulting and Clinical Psychology, 75*(6), 842–852.

Ball, S. A., Martino, S., Nich, C., Frankforter, T. L., van Horn, D., Crits-Christoph, P., . . . Carroll, K. M. (2007). Site matters: Multisite randomized trial of motivational enhancement therapy in community drug abuse clinics. *Journal of Consulting and Clinical Psychology, 75*, 556–567.

Bamatter, W., Carroll, K. M., Añez, L. M., Paris, M. J., Ball, S. A., Nich, C., . . . Martino, S. (2010). Informal discussions in substance abuse treatment sessions with Spanish-speaking clients. *Journal of Substance Abuse Treatment, 39*(4), 353–363.

Bandura, A. (1982). Self-efficacy mechanism in human agency. *American Psychologist, 37*, 122–147.

Bandura, A. (1986). *Social foundations of thought and action: A social cognitive theory.* Englewood Cliffs, NJ: Prentice-Hall.

Bandura, A. (1997). *Self-efficacy: The exercise of control.* New York: Freeman.

Barlow, D. H. (Ed.). (2014). *Clinical handbook of psychological disorders: A step-by-step treatment manual* (5th ed.). New York: Guilford Press.

Barnicot, K., Wampold, B., & Priebe, S. (2014). The effect of core clinician interpersonal behaviours on depression. *Journal of Affective Disorders, 167,* 112–117.

Barrett-Lennard, G. T. (1962). Dimensions of therapist response as causal factors in therapeutic change. *Psychological Monographs: General and Applied, 76*(43), 1–36.

Barrett-Lennard, G. T. (1981). The empathy cycle: Refinement of a nuclear concept. *Journal of Counseling Psychology, 28*(2), 91–100.

Barry, M. J., & Edgman-Levitan, S. (2012). Shared decision making—Pinnacle of patient-centered care. *New England Journal of Medicine, 366*(9), 780–781.

Batson, C. D., Klein, T. R., Highberger, L., & Shaw, L. L. (1995). Immorality from empathy-induced altruism: When compassion and justice conflict. *Journal of Personality and Social Psychology, 68*(6), 1042–1054.

Battersby, M., Von Korff, M., Schaefer, J., Davis, C., Ludman, E., Greene, S. M., . . . Wagner, E. H. (2010). Twelve evidence-based principles for implementing self-management support in primary care. *Joint Commission Journal on Quality and Patient Safety, 36*(12), 561–570.

Beidas, R. S., & Kendall, P. C. (2010). Training therapists in evidence-based practice: A critical review of studies from a systems-contextual perspective. *Clinical Psychology: Science and Practice, 17*(1), 1–30.

Bellg, A., Borrelli, B., Resnick, B., Ogedegbe, G., Hecht, J., Ernst, D., & Czajkowski, S. (2004). Enhancing treatment fidelity in health behavior change studies: Best practices and recommendations from the Behavioral Change Consortium. *Health Psychology, 23*(5), 443–451.

Bem, D. J. (1967). Self-perception: An alternative interpretation of cognitive dissonance phenomena. *Psychological Review, 74,* 183–200.

Bem, D. J. (1972). Self-perception theory. In L. Berkowitz (Ed.), *Advances in experimental social psychology* (Vol. 6, pp. 1–62). New York: Academic Press.

Benson, H., & Klipper, M. Z. (2000). *The relaxation response.* New York: Quill.

Berg, I. K., & Reuss, N. H. (1997). *Solutions step by step: A substance abuse treatment manual.* New York: Norton.

Bernstein, J., Bernstein, E., Tassiopoulos, K., Heeren, T., Levenson, S., & Hingson, R. (2005). Brief motivational intervention at a clinic visit reduces cocaine and heroin use. *Drug and Alcohol Dependence, 77,* 49–59.

Bertholet, N., Faouzi, M., Gmel, G., Gaume, J., & Daeppen, J. B. (2010). Change talk sequence during brief motivational intervention, towards or away from drinking. *Addiction, 105,* 2106–2112.

Beutler, L. E., Harwood, T. M., Michelson, A., Song, X., & Holman, J. (2011). Resistance/reactance level. *Journal of Clinical Psychology: In Session, 67*(2), 133–142.

Beutler, L. E., Kimpara, S., Edwards, C. J., & Miller, K. D. (2018). Fitting psychotherapy to patient coping style: A meta-analysis. *Journal of Clinical Psychology, 74*(11), 1980–1995.

Beutler, L. E., Machado, P. P. P., & Neufeldt, S. A. (1994). Therapist variables. In A. E. Bergin & S. L. Garfield (Eds.), *Handbook of psychotherapy and behavior change* (4th ed., pp. 229–269). New York: Wiley.

Bien, T. H., Miller, W. R., & Boroughs, J. M. (1993). Motivational interviewing with alcohol outpatients. *Behavioural and Cognitive Psychotherapy, 21,* 347–356.

Bien, T. H., Miller, W. R., & Tonigan, J. S. (1993). Brief interventions for alcohol problems: A review. *Addiction, 88,* 315–336.

Bischoff, M. M., & Tracey, T. J. G. (1995). Client resistance as predicted by therapist behavior: A study of sequential dependence. *Journal of Consulting and Clinical Psychology, 42*(4), 487–495.

Bloom, P. (2016). *Against empathy: The case for rational compassion.* New York: HarperCollins.

Blow, A. J., Sprenkle, D. H., & Davis, S. D. (2007). Is who delivers the treatment more important than the treatment itself?: The role of the therapist in common factors. *Journal of Marital and Family Therapy, 33*(3), 298–317.

Bohart, A. C., & Tallman, K. (1999). *How clients make therapy work: The process of active self-healing.* Washington, DC: American Psychological Association.

Bohart, A. C., & Tallman, K. (2010). Clients: The neglected common factor in psychotherapy. In B. L. Duncan, S. D. Miller, B. E. Wampold, & M. A. Hubble (Eds.), *The heart and soul of change: Delivering what works in therapy* (2nd ed., pp. 83–112). Washington, DC: American Psychological Association.

Boswell, J. F., Gallagher, M. W., Sauer-Zavala, S. E., Bullis, J., Gorman, J. M., Shear, M. K., . . . Barlow, D. H. (2013). Patient characteristics and variability in adherence and competence in cognitive-behavioral therapy for panic disorder. *Journal of Consulting and Clinical Psychology, 81*(3), 443–454.

Bozarth, J. D. (1984). Beyond reflection: Emergent modes of empathy. In R. F. Levant & J. M. Shlien (Eds.), *Client-centered therpy and the person-centered approach: New directions in theory, research, and practice.* (pp. 59–75). Westport, CT: Praeger/Greenwood.

Brehm, J. W. (1966). *A theory of psychological reactance.* New York: Academic Press.

Brehm, S. S., & Brehm, J. W. (1981). *Psychological reactance: A theory of freedom and control.* New York: Academic Press.

Brooks, D. (2015). *The road to character.* New York: Random House.

Brown, G. S., Lambert, M. J., Jones, E. R., & Minami, T. (2005). Identifying highly effective psychotherapists in a managed care environment. *American Journal of Managed Care, 11*(8), 513–520.

Brown, J., & Miller, W. R. (1993). Impact of motivational interviewing on participation and outcome in residential alcoholism treatment. *Psychology of Addictive Behaviors, 7,* 211–218.

Brown, K. W., Ryan, R. M., & Creswell, J. D. (2007). Mindfulness: Theoretical foundations and evidence for its salutary effects. *Psychological Inquiry, 18*(4), 211–237.

Budge, S. L., Owen, J. J., Kopta, S. M., Minami, T., Hanson, M. R., & Hirsch, G. (2013). Differences among trainees in client outcomes associated with the phase model of change. *Psychotherapy, 50*(2), 150–157.

Bugental, J. (1999). *Psychotherapy isn't what you think: Bringing the psychotherapeutic engagement into the living moment.* Phoenix, AZ: Zeig, Tucker & Co.

Burns, D. D., & Nolen-Hoeksma, S. (1992). Therapeutic empathy and recovery from depression in cognitive-behavioral therapy: A structural equation model. *Journal of Consulting and Clinical Psychology, 60*(3), 441–449.

Burwell-Pender, L., & Halinski, K. H. (2008). Enhanced awareness of countertransference. *Journal of Professional Counseling: Practice, Theory and Research, 36*(2).

Campbell, A. N. C., Turrigiano, E., Moore, M., Miele, G. M., Rieckmann, T., Hu, M.-C., . . . Nunes, E. V. (2015). Acceptability of a Web-based community reinforcement approach for substance use disorders with treatment-seeking American Indians/Alaska Natives. *Community Mental Health Journal, 51*(4), 393–403.

Campbell, B. K., Guydish, J., Le, T., Wells, E. A., & McCarty, D. (2015). The relationship of therapeutic alliance and treatment delivery fidelity with treatment retention in a multisite trial of twelve-step facilitation. *Psychology of Addictive Behaviors, 29*(1), 106–113.

Campbell, R. G., & Babrow, A. S. (2004). The role of empathy in responses to persuasive risk communication: Overcoming resistance to HIV prevention messages. *Health Communication, 16*(2), 159–182.

Campbell, S. D., Adamson, S. J., & Carter, J. D. (2010). Client language during motivational enhancement therapy and alcohol use outcome. *Behavioural and Cognitive Psychotherapy, 38*(4), 399–415.

Campinez Navarro, M., Perula de Torres, L. A., Bosch Fontcuberta, J. M., Barragan Brun, N., Arbonies Ortiz, J. C., Novo Rodriguez, J. M., . . . Romero Rodriguez, E. M. (2016). Measuring the quality of motivational interviewing in primary health care encounters: The development and validation of the Motivational Interviewing Assessment Scale (MIAS). *European Journal of General Practice, 22*(3), 182–188.

Carkhuff, R. R. (2019). *The art of helping* (10th ed.). Amherst, MA: HRD Press.

Carkhuff, R. R., & Truax, C. B. (1965). Training in counseling and psychotherapy: An evaluation of an integrated didactic and experiential approach. *Journal of Consulting Psychology, 29*, 333–336.

Carroll, K. M. (1998). *A cognitive-behavioral approach: Treating cocaine addiction*. Rockville, MD: National Instsitute on Drug Abuse.

Carroll, K. M., Connors, G. J., Cooney, N. L., DiClemente, C. C., Donovan, D. M., Kadden, R. R., . . . Zweben, A. (1998). Internal validity of Project MATCH treatments: Discriminability and integrity. *Journal of Consulting and Clinical Psychology, 66*(2), 290–303.

Castonguay, L. G., Boswell, J. F., Constantino, M. J., Goldfried, M. R., & Hill, C. E. (2010). Training implications of harmful effects of psychological treatments. *American Psychologist, 65*(1), 34–49.

Castonguay, L. G., Goldfried, M. R., Wiser, S., Raue, P. J., & Hayes, A. M. (1996). Predicting the effect of cognitive therapy for depression: A study of unique and common factors. *Journal of Consulting and Clinical Psychology, 64*(3), 497–504.

Chamberlain, P., Patterson, G., Reid, J., Kavanagh, K., & Forgatch, M. S. (1984). Observation of client resistance. *Behavior Therapy, 15*, 144–155.

Chambless, D. L., Baker, M. J., Baucom, D. H., Beutler, L. E., Calhoun, K. S., Crits-Christoph, P., . . . Woody, S. R. (1998). Update on empirically validated therapies: II. *Clinical Psychologist, 51*(1), 3–16.

Chambless, D. L., & Ollendick, T. H. (2001). Empirically supported psychological interventions: Controversies and evidence. *Annual Review of Clinical Psychology, 52*, 685–716.

Cheavens, J. S., Feldman, J. S., Woodward, J. T., & Snyder, C. R. (2006). Hope in cognitive psychotherapies: On working with client strengths. *Journal of Cognitive Psychotherapy, 20*(2), 135–145.

Chick, J., Ritson, B., Connaughton, J., & Stewart, A. (1988). Advice versus extended treatment for alcoholism: a controlled study. *British Journal of Addiction, 83*(2), 159–170.

Chow, D. L., Miller, S. D., Seidel, J. A., Kane, R. T., Thornton, J. A., & Andrews, W. P. (2015). The role of deliberate practice in the development of highly effective psychotherapists. *Psychotherapy, 52*(3), 337–345.

Coco, G. L., Gullo, S., Prestano, C., & Gelso, C. J. (2011). Relation of the real relationship and the working alliance to the outcome of brief psychotherapy. *Psychotherapy, 48*(4), 359–367.

Collins, N. L., & Miller, L. C. (1994). Self-disclosure and liking: A meta-analytic review. *Psychological Bulletin, 116*(3), 457–475.

Colosimo, K. A., & Pos, A. E. (2015). A rational model of expressed therapeutic presence. *Journal of Psychotherapy Integration, 25*(2), 100–114.

Constantino, M. J., Glass, C. R., Arnkoff, D. B., Ametrano, R. M., & Smith, J. Z. (2011). Expectations. In J. C. Norcross (Ed.), *Psychotherapy relationships that work: Evidence-based responsiveness* (pp. 354–376). New York: Oxford University Press.

Critcher, C. R., Dunning, D., & Armor, D. A. (2010). When self-affirmations reduce defensiveness: Timing is key. *Personality and Social Psychology Bulletin, 36*(7), 947–959.

Critchley, H. D. (2009). Psychophysiology of neural, cognitive and affective integration: fMRI and autonomic indicants. *International Journal of Psychophysiology, 73*(2), 88–94.

Crits-Christoph, P., Baranackie, K., Kurcias, J. S., & Beck, A. T. (1991). Meta-analysis of therapist effects in psychotherapy outcome studies. *Psychotherapy Research, 1*(2), 81–91.

Crits-Christoph, P., Frank, E., Chambless, D. L., Brody, C., & Karp, J. F. (1995). Training in empirically validated treatments: What are clinical psychology students learning? *Professional Psychology: Research and Practice, 26*, 514–522.

Daeppen, J.-B., Bertholet, N., Gmel, G., & Gaume, J. (2007). Communication during brief intervention, intention to change, and outcome. *Substance Abuse, 28*(3), 43–51.

Dalai Lama, The, & Hopkins, J. (2017). *The heart of meditation: Discovering innermost awareness.* Boulder, CO: Shambala Books.

Dalai Lama, The, & Vreeland, N. (2001). *An open heart: Practicing compassion in everyday life.* New York: Little, Brown.

Davis, D. M., & Hayes, J. A. (2011). What are the benefits of mindfulness?: A practice review of psychotherapy-related research. *Psychotherapy, 48*(2), 198–208.

Davison, G. C., Vogel, R. S., & Coffman, S. G. (1997). Think-aloud approaches to cognitive assessment and the articulated thoughts in simulated situations paradigm. *Journal of Consulting and Clinical Psychology, 65*(6), 950–958.

Dawes, R. M. (1994). *House of cards.* New York: Free Press.

de Almeida Neto, A. C. (2017). Understanding motivational interviewing: An evolutionary perspective. *Evolutionary Psychological Science, 3*(4), 379–389.

Deci, E. L., Koestner, R., & Ryan, R. M. (1999). A meta-analytic review of experiments examining the effects of extrinsic rewards on intrinsic motivation. *Psychological Bulletin, 125*(6), 627–668.

Deci, E. L., & Ryan R. M. (2008). Self-determination theory: A macrotheory of human motivation, development, and health. *Canadian Psychology, 49*(3), 182–185.

Decker, S. E., Carroll, K. M., Nich, C., Canning-Ball, M., & Martino, S. (2013). Correspondence of motivational interviewing adherence and competence ratings in real and role-played client sessions. *Psychological Assessment, 25*(1), 306–312.

DeJonge, J. J. M., Schippers, G. M., & Schaap, C. P. D. R. (2005). The Motivational Interviewing Skill Code: Reliability and a critical appraisal. *Behavioural and Cognitive Psychotherapy, 33*, 1–14.

Delaney, H. D., & DiClemente, C. C. (2005). Psychology's roots: A brief history of the influence of Judeo-Christian perspectives. In W. R. Miller & H. D. Delaney (Eds.), *Judeo-Christian perspectives on psychology: Human nature, motivation, and change* (pp. 31–54). Washington, DC: American Psychological Association.

Delaney, H. D., Miller, W. R., & Bisonó, A. M. (2007). Religiosity and spirituality among psychologists: A survey of clinician members of the American Psychological Association. *Professional Psychology: Research and Practice, 38*(5), 538–546.

Deming, W. E. (2000). *The new economics for industry, government, education* (2nd ed.). Cambridge, MA: MIT Press.

deShazer, S., Dolan, Y., Korman, H., Trepper, T., McCollum, E., & Berg, I. K. (2007). *More than miracles: The state of the art of solution-focused brief therapy*. Binghamton, NY: Haworth Press.

DeVargas, E. C., & Stormshak, E. A. (2020). Motivational interviewing skills as predictors of change in emerging adult risk behavior. *Professional Psychology: Research and Practice, 51*(1), 16–24.

Di Bartolomeo, A. A., Shukla, S., Westra, H. A., Ghashghaei, N. S., & Olson, D. S. (in press). Rolling with resistance: A client language analysis of deliberate practice in continuing education for psychotherapists. *Counselling and Psychotherpy Research*.

DiClemente, C. C. (2003). *Addiction and change: How addictions develop and addicted people recover*. New York: Guilford Press.

DiClemente, C. C., Corno, C. M., Graydon, M. M., Wiprovnick, A. E., & Knoblach, D. J. (2017). Motivational interviewing, enhancement, and brief interventions over the last decade: A review of reviews of efficacy and effectiveness. *Psychology of Addictive Behaviors, 31*(8), 862–887.

Dillard, J. P., & Shen, L. (2005). On the nature of reactance and its role in persuasive health communication. *Communication Monographs, 72*(2), 144–168.

Dimidjian, S., & Hollon, S. D. (2010). How would we know if psychotherapy were harmful? *American Psychologist, 65*(1), 21–33.

Drage, L., Masterson, C., Tober, G., Farragher, T., & Bewick, B. (2019). The impact of therapists' responses to resistance to change: A sequential analysis of therapist–client interactions in motivational interviewing. *Alcohol and Alcoholism, 54*(2), 173–176.

Duan, C., & Hill, C. E. (1996). The current state of empathy research. *Journal of Counseling Psychology, 43*(3), 261–274.

Duncan, B. L., Miller, S. D., Wampold, B. E., & Hubble, M. A. (Eds.). (2010). *The heart and soul of change: Delivering what works in therapy* (2nd ed.). Washington, DC: American Psychological Association.

Edwards, C. J., Beutler, L. E., & Someah, K. (2019). Reactance level. In J. C. Norcross & B. E. Wampold (Eds.), *Psychotherapy relationships that work: Vol. 2. Evidence-based therapist responsiveness* (pp. 188–211). New York: Oxford University Press.

Edwards, G., & Orford, J. (1977). A plain treatment for alcoholism. *Proceedings of the Royal Society of Medicine, 70*(5), 344–348.

Edwards, G., Orford, J., Egert, S., Guthrie, S., Hawker, A., Hensman, C., . . . Taylor, C. (1977). Alcoholism: A controlled trial of "treatment" and "advice." *Journal of Studies on Alcohol, 38*, 1004–1031.

Egan, G. (2014). *The skilled helper: A problem-management and opportunity-development approach to helping* (10th ed.). Belmont, CA: Brooks/Cole Cengage Learning.

Elkin, I., Falconnier, L., Smith, Y., Canada, K. E., Henderson, E., Brown, E. R., & McKay, B. M. (2014). Therapist responsiveness and patient engagement in therapy. *Psychotherapy Research: Journal of the Society for Psychotherapy Research, 24*(1), 52–66.

Elliott, R., Bohart, A. C., Watson, J. C., & Greenberg, L. S. (2011a). Empathy. In J. C. Norcross (Ed.), *Psychotherapy relationships that work: Evidence-based responsiveness* (pp. 132–152). New York: Oxford Unversity Press.

Elliott, R., Bohart, A. C., Watson, J. C., & Greenberg, L. S. (2011b). Empathy. *Psychotherapy, 48*(1), 43–49.

Elliott, R., Bohart, A. C., Watson, J. C., & Murphy, D. (2018). Therapist empathy and client outcome: An updated meta-analysis. *Psychotherapy, 55*(4), 399–410.

Ellis, J. D., Grekin, E. R., Beatty, J. R., McGoron, L., LaLiberte, B. V., Pop, D. E., . . . Ondersma, S. J. (2017). Effects of narrator empathy in a computer delivered brief intervention for alcohol use. *Contemporary Clinical Trials, 61,* 29–32.

Ellis, M. V., Berger, L., Hanus, A. E., Ayala, E. E., Swords, B. A., & Siembor, M. (2014). Inadequate and harmful clinical supervision: Testing a revised framework and assessing occurrence. *Counseling Psychologist, 42*(4), 434–472.

Elwyn, G., Dehlendorf, C., Epstein, R. M., Marrin, K., White, J., & Frosch, D.L. (2014). Shared decision making and motivational interviewing: Achieving patient-centered care across the spectrum of health care problems. *Annals of Family Medicine, 12*(3), 270–275.

Elwyn, G., & Frosch, D. L. (2016). Shared decision making and motivational interviewing: Achieving patient-centered care across the spectrum of health care problems. *Annals of Family Medicine, 12*(3), 270–275.

Engle, D., & Arkowitz, H. (2006). *Ambivalence in psychotherapy: Facilitating readiness to change.* New York: Guilford Press.

Epton, T., Harris, P. R., Kane, R., van Konigsbruggen, G. M., & Sheeran, P. (2015). The impact of self-affirmation on health-behavior change: A meta-analysis. *Health Psychology, 34*(3), 187–196.

Erekson, D. M., Clayson, R., Park, S. Y., & Tass, S. (2020). Therapist effects on early change in psychotherapy in a naturalistic setting. *Psychotherapy Research, 30*(1), 68–78.

Erekson, D. M., Janis, R., Bailey, R. J., Cattani, K., & Pedersen, T. R. (2017). A longitudinal investigation of the impact of psychotherapist training: Does training improve client outcomes? *Journal of Counseling Psychology, 64*(5), 514–524.

Ericsson, K. A., Krampe, R. T., & Tesch-Römer, C. (1993). The role of deliberate practice in the acquisition of expert performance. *Psychological Review, 100*(3), 363–406.

Ericsson, K. A., & Pool, R. (2016). *Peak: Secrets from the new science of expertise.* Boston: Houghton Mifflin Harcourt.

Eubanks, C. F., Muran, J. C., & Safran, J. D. (2018). Alliance rupture repair: A meta-analysis. *Psychotherapy, 55*(4), 508–519.

Eubanks-Carter, C., Muran, J. C., & Safran, J. D. (2015). Alliance-focused training. *Psychotherapy, 52*(2), 169–173.

Falkenström, F., Markowitz, J. C., Jonker, H., Philips, B., & Holmqvist, R. (2013). Can psychotherapists function as their own controls?: Meta-analysis of the "crossed therapist" design in comparative psychotherapy trials. *Journal of Clinical Psychiatry, 74*(5), 482–491.

Farber, B. A. (2006). *Self-disclosure in psychotherapy.* New York: Guilford Press.

Farber, B. A., & Doolin, E. M. (2011a). Positive regard. *Psychotherapy, 48*(1), 58–64.

Farber, B. A., & Doolin, E. M. (2011b). Positive regard and affirmation. In J. C.

Norcross (Ed.), *Psychotherapy relationships that work* (2nd ed., pp. 168–186). New York: Oxford University Press.

Farber, B. A., Suzuki, J. Y., & Lynch, D. A. (2018). Positive regard and psychotherapy outcome: A meta-analytic review. *Psychotherapy, 55*(4), 411–423.

Ferster, C. B., & Skinner, B. F. (1957). *Schedules of reinforcement.* Englewood Cliffs, NJ: Prentice-Hall.

Festinger, L. (1957). *A theory of cognitive dissonance.* Stanford, CA: Stanford University Press.

Finley, J. (2020). *Turning to the Mystics: Thomas Merton.* Retrieved from *https://cac.org/podcast/turning-to-the-mystics.*

Fischer, D. J., & Moyers, T. B. (2014). Is there an association between empathic speech and change talk in motivational interviewing sessions? *Alcoholism Treatment Quarterly, 32*(1), 3–18.

Fixsen, D. L., Blase, K. A., & Van Dyke, M. K. (2019). *Implementation practice and science.* Chapel Hill, NC: Active Implementation Research Network.

Fixsen, D. L., Naoom, S. F., Blase, K. A., Friedman, R. M., & Wallace, F. (2005). *Implementation research: A synthesis of the literature.* Tampa: University of South Florida, National Implementation Research Network.

Flückiger, C., Del Re, A. C., Wlodasch, D., Horvath, A. O., Solomonov, N., & Wampold, B. E. (in press). Assessing the alliance–outcome association adjusted for patient characteristics and treatment processes: A meta-analytic summary of direct comparisons. *Journal of Counseling Psychology.*

Fonagy, P., Gergely, G., & Jurist, E. L. (Eds.). (2002). *Affect regulation, mentalization and the development of self.* New York: Other Press.

Ford, M. E. (1992). *Motivating humans: Goals, emotions, and personal agency beliefs.* Newbury Park, CA: SAGE.

Forrester, D., Westlake, D., Killian, M., Antonopolou, V., McCann, M., Thurnham, A., . . . Hutchison, D. (2019). What is the relationship between worker skills and outcomes for families in child and family social work. *British Journal of Social Work, 49,* 2148–2167.

Fox, T. (2017). *Therapists' observations of quantum change among clients with drug and alcohol dependency: A thematic analysis.* Doctoral dissertation, University of Leicester, Leicester, UK.

Frank, J. D. (1968). The role of hope in psychotherapy. *International Journal of Psychiatry, 5*(5), 383–395.

Frank, J. D. (1971). Therapeutic factors in psychotherapy. *American Journal of Psychotherapy, 25*(3), 350–361.

Frank, J. D., & Frank, J. B. (1993). *Persuasion and healing: A comparative study of psychotherapy* (3rd ed.). Baltimore: Johns Hopkins University Press.

Frankl, V. E. (2006). *Man's search for meaning.* Boston: Beacon Press.

Franklin, B. (1785). *Report of Dr. Benjamin Franklin, and other commissioners, charged by the King of France, with the examination of the animal magnetism, as now practiced in Paris.* London: J. Johnson.

Franklin, B. (2012/1785). *The art of virtue.* New York: Skyhorse.

French, D. P., Olander, E. K., Chisholm, A., & McSharry, J. (2014). Which behaviour change techniques are most effective at increasing older adults' self-efficacy and physical activity behavior?: A systematic review. *Annals of Behavioral Medicine, 48*(2), 225–234.

Fromm, E. (1956). *The art of loving.* New York: Bantam.

Gallese, V., Gernsbacher, M. A., Heyes, C., Hickok, G., & Iacoboni, M. (2011). Mirror neuron forum. *Perspectives on Psychological Science, 6*(4), 369–407.

Gaume, J., Bertholet, N., Faouzi, M., Gmel, G., & Daeppen, J. B. (2010). Counselor motivational interviewing skills and young adult change talk articulation during brief motivational interventions. *Journal of Substance Abuse Treatment, 39*(3), 272–281.

Gaume, J., Gmel, G., Faouzi, M., & Daeppen, J. B. (2009). Counselor skill influences outcomes of brief motivational interventions. *Journal of Substance Abuse Treatment, 37*(2), 151–159.

Geller, S. M., & Greenberg, L. S. (2018). *Therapeutic presence: A mindful approach to effective therapy.* Washington, DC: American Psychological Association.

Gelso, C. J., & Carter, J. A. (1994). Components of the psychotherapy relationship: Their interaction and unfolding during treatment. *Journal of Counseling Psychology, 41*(3), 296–306.

Gelso, C. J., & Kanninen, K. M. (2017). Neutrality revisited: On the value of being neutral within an empathic atmosphere. *Journal of Psychotherapy Integration, 27*(3), 330–341.

Gelso, C. J., Kivlighan, D. M., Busa-Knepp, J., Spiegel, E. B., Ain, S., Hummel, A. M., . . . Markin, R. D. (2012). The unfolding of the real relationship and the outcome of brief psychotherapy. *Journal of Counseling Psychology, 59*(4), 495–506.

Gelso, C. J., Kivlighan, D. M., & Markin, R. D. (2018). The real relationship and its role in psychotherapy outcome: A meta-analysis. *Psychotherapy, 55*(4), 434–444.

Gelso, C. J., & Perez-Rojas, A. E. (2017). Inner experience and the good therapist. In L. G. Castonguay & C. E. Hill (Eds.), *How and why are some therapists better than others?: Understanding therapist effects* (pp. 101–115). Washington, DC: American Psychological Association.

Gendlin, E. T. (1961). Experiencing: A variable in the process of therapeutic change. *American Journal of Psychotherapy, 15*(2), 233–245.

Ghaderi, A. (2006). Does individualization matter?: A randomized trial of standardized (focused) versus individualized (broad) cognitive behavior therapy for bulimia nervosa. *Behaviour Research and Therapy, 44*(2), 273–288.

Giannini, H. C. (2017). Hope as grounds for forgiveness: A Christian argument for universal, unconditional forgiveness. *Journal of Religious Ethics, 45*(1), 58–82.

Gillberg, C. (1996). The long-term outcome of childhood empathy disorders. *European Child and Adolescent Psychiatry, 5*, 52–56.

Gist, M. E., & Mitchell, T. R. (1992). Self-efficacy: A theoretical analysis of its determinants and malleability. *Academy of Management Review, 17*(2), 183–211.

Gladwell, M. (2008). *Outliers: The story of success.* New York: Little, Brown.

Glynn, L. H., & Moyers, T. B. (2010). Chasing change talk: The clinician's role in evoking client language about change. *Journal of Substance Abuse Treatment, 39*(1), 65–70.

Godley, S. H., Meyers, R. J., Smith, J. E., Karvinen, T., Titus, J. C., Godley, M. D., . . . Kelberg, P. (2001). *The adolescent community reinforcement approach for adolescent cannabis users* (Vol. 4). Rockville, MD: Center for Substance Abuse Treatment.

Goldberg, S. B., Babins-Wagner, R., & Miller, S. D. (2017). Nurturing expertise at mental health agencies. In T. Rousmaniere, R. K. Goodyear, S. D. Miller, & B. E. Wampold (Eds.), *The cycle of excellence: Using deliberate practice to improve supervision and training* (pp. 199–217). Hoboken, NJ: Wiley.

Goldberg, S. B., Hoyt, W. T., Nissen-Lie, H. A., Nielsen, S. L., & Wampold, B.

E. (2018). Unpacking the therapist effect: Impact of treatment length differs for high- and low-performing therapists. *Psychotherapy Research, 28*(4), 532–544.

Goldberg, S. B., Rousmaniere, T., Miller, S. D., Whipple, J., Nielsen, S. V., Hoyt, W. T., & Wampold, B. E. (2016). Do psychotherapists improve with time and experience?: A longitudinal analysis of outcomes in a clinical setting. *Journal of Counseling Psychology, 63*(1), 1–11.

Goldman, R. N., Greenberg, L. S., & Pos, A. E. (2005). Depth of emotional experience and outcome. *Psychotherapy Research, 15*(3), 248–260.

Goldstein, A. P., & Shipman, W. G. (1961). Patients' expectancies, symptom reduction and aspects of he initial psychotherapeutic interview. *Journal of Clinical Psychology, 17,* 129–133.

Gollwitzer, P. M. (1999). Implementation intentions: Simple effects of simple plans. *American Psychologist, 54*(7), 493–503.

Gollwitzer, P. M., Wieber, F., Myers, A. L., & McCrea, S. M. (2010). How to maximize implementation intention effects. In C. R. Agnew, D. E. Carlston, W. G. Graziano, & J. R. Kelly (Eds.), *Then a miracle occurs: Focusing on behavior in social psychological theory and research* (pp. 137–161). New York: Oxford University Press.

Gordon, T. (1970). *Parent effectiveness training.* New York: Wyden.

Gordon, T., & Edwards, W. S. (1997). *Making the patient your partner: Communication skills for doctors and other caregivers.* New York: Auburn House.

Gorman, D. M. (2017). Has the National Registry of Evidence-Based Programs and Practices (NREPP) lost its way? *International Journal of Drug Policy, 45,* 40–41.

Gotink, R. A., Chu, P., Busschbach, J. J. V., Benson, H., Fricchione, G. L., & Hunink, M. (2015). Standardized mindfulness-based interventions in healthcare: An overview of systematic reviews and meta-analyses of RCTd. *PLOS ONE, 10*(4), e0124344.

Grafanaki, S. (2001). What counselling research has taught us about the concept of congruence: Main discoveries and unsolved issues. In G. Wyatt (Ed.), *Congruence* (pp. 18–35). Monmouth, UK: PCCS Books.

Greenberg, L. S., & Elliott, R. (1997). Varieties of empathic responding. In A. C. Bohart & L. S. Greenberg (Eds.), *Empathy reconsidered: New directions in psychotherapy* (pp. 167–186). Washington, DC: American Psychological Association.

Greenberg, L. S., & Geller, S. (2001). Congruence and therapeutic presence. In G. Wyatt (Ed.), *Rogers' therapeutic conditions: Evolution, theory and practice: Vol. 1. Congruence* (pp. 131–149). Ross-on-Wye, UK: PCCS Books.

Haley, J. (1993). *Uncommon therapy: The psychiatric techniques of Milton H. Erickson.* New York: Norton.

Hall, K., Staiger, P. K., Simpson, A., Best, D., & Lubman, D. I. (2016). After 30 years of dissemination, have we achieved sustained practice change in motivational interviewing? *Addiction, 111*(7), 1144–1150.

Hannover, W., Blaut, C., Kniehase, C., Martin, T., & Hannich, H. J. (2013). Interobserver agreement of the German translation of the Motivational Interviewing Sequential Code for Observing Process Exchanges (MI-SCOPE;D). *Psychology of Addictive Behaviors, 27*(4), 1196–1200.

Harris, K. B., & Miller, W. R. (1990). Behavioral self-control training for problem drinkers: Components of efficacy. *Psychology of Addictive Behaviors, 4,* 82–90.

Hatcher, R. L. (2015). Interpersonal competencies: Responsiveness, technique, and training in psychotherapy. *American Psychologist, 70*(8), 747–757.

Haug, T., Nordgreen, T., Öst, L.-G., Tangen, T., Kvale, G., Hovland, O. J., . . . Havik, O. E. (2016). Working alliance and competence as predictors of outcome in cognitive behavioral therapy for social anxiety and panic disorder in adults. *Behaviour Research and Therapy, 77,* 40–51.

Hayes, J. A., Gelso, C. J., & Hummel, A. M. (2011). Managing countertransference. *Psychotherapy, 48*(1), 88–97.

Hayes, S. C. (2004). Acceptance and commitment therapy, relational frame theory, and the third wave of behavioral and cognitive therapies. *Behavior Therapy, 35*(4), 639–665.

Hayes, S. C., Lafollette, V. M., & Linehan, M. M. (Eds.). (2011). *Mindfulness and accceptance: Expanding the cognitive-behavioral tradition.* New York: Guilford Press.

Henggeler, S. W., Melton, G. B., Brondino, M. J., Scherer, D. G., & Hanley, J. H. (1997). Multisystemic therapy with violent and chronic juvenile offenders and their families: The role of treatment fidelity in successful dissemination. *Journal of Consulting and Clinical Psychology, 65*(5), 821–833.

Henggeler, S. W., Schoenwald, S. K., Letourneau, J. G., & Edwards, D. L. (2002). Transporting efficacious treatments to field settings: The link between supervisory practices and therapist fidelity in MST programs. *Journal of Clinical Child and Adolescent Psychology, 31,* 155–167.

Henretty, J. R., Currier, J. M., Berman, J. S., & Levitt, H. M. (2014). The impact of counselor self-disclosure on clients: A meta-analytic review of experimental and quasi-experimental research. *Journal of Counseling Psychology, 61*(2), 191–207.

Herschell, A. D., Kolko, D. J., Baumann, B. L., & Davis, A. C. (2010). The role of therapist training in the implementation of psychosocial treatments: A review and critique with recommendations. *Clinical Psychology Review, 30*(4), 448–466.

Hersoug, A. G., Hoglend, P., Monsen, J. T., & Havik, O. E. (2001). Quality of working alliance in psychotherapy: Therapist variables and patient/therapist similarity as predictors. *Journal of Psychotherapy Practice and Research, 10*(4), 205–216.

Hettema, J., Steele, J., & Miller, W. R. (2005). Motivational interviewing. *Annual Review of Clinical Psychology, 1,* 91–111.

Hill, C. E. (1990). Exploratory in-session process research in individual psychotherapy: A review. *Journal of Consulting and Clinical Psychology, 58*(3), 288–294.

Hill, C. E. (2005). Therapist techniques, client involvement, and the therapeutic relationship: Inextricably intertwined in the therapy process. *Psychotherapy: Theory, Research and Practice, 42*(4), 431–442.

Hill, C. E., Helms, J. E., Tichenor, V., Spiegel, S. B., O'Grady, K. E., & Perry, E. S. (1988). Effects of therapist response modes in brief psychotherapy. *Journal of Counseling Psychology, 35*(3), 222–233.

Hill, C. E., & Knox, S. (2013). Training and supervision. In M. J. Lambert (Ed.), *Bergin and Garfield's handbook of psychotherapy and behavior change* (6th ed., pp. 775–811). Hoboken, NJ: Wiley.

Hill, C. E., Knox, S., & Pinto-Coelho, K. G. (2018). Therapist self-disclosure and immediacy: A qualitative meta-analysis. *Psychotherapy, 55*(4), 445–460.

Hill, C. E., O'Grady, K. E., & Elkin, I. (1992). Applying the Collaborative Study Psychotherapy Rating Scale to rate therapist adherence in cognitive-behavior therapy, interpersonal therapy, and clinical management. *Journal of Consulting and Clinical Psychology, 60*(1), 73–79.

Hofmann, S. G., & Barlow, D. H. (2014). Evidence-based psychological interventions and the common factors approach: The beginnings of a rapprochement? *Psychotherapy, 51*(4), 510–513.

Hojat, M. (2007). *Empathy in patient care: Antecedents, development, measurement and outcomes.* New York: Springer.

Holländare, F., Gustafsson, S. A., Berglind, M., Grape, F., Carlbring, P., Andersson, G, . . . Tillfors, M. (2016). Therapist behaviours in internet-based cognitive behaviour therapy (ICBT) for depressive symptoms. *Internet Interventions, 3,* 1–7.

Hood, R. W., Jr., Hill, P. C., & Spilka, B. (2018). *The psychology of religion: An empirical approach* (5th ed.). New York: Guilford Press.

Horvath, A. O. (2000). The therapeutic relationship: From transference to alliance. *Journal of Clinical Psychology, 56*(2), 163–173.

Horvath, A. O., Del Re, A. C., Flückinger, C., & Symonds, D. (2011). Alliance in individual psychotherapy. *Psychotherapy, 48*(1), 9–16.

Horvath, A. O., & Greenberg, L. S. (1994). *The working alliance: Theory, research, and practice.* New York: Wiley.

Houck, J. M., Manuel, J. K., & Moyers, T. B. (2018). Short- and long-term effects of within-session client speech on drinking outcomes in the COMBINE study. *Journal of Studies on Alcohol and Drugs, 79*(2), 217–222.

Howe, L. C., Goyer, J. P., & Crum, A. J. (2017). Harnessing the placebo effect: Exploring the infuence of physician characteristics on placebo response. *Health Psychology, 36*(11), 1074–1082.

Hunt, G. M., & Azrin, N. H. (1973). A community-reinforcement approach to alcoholism. *Behaviour Research and Therapy, 11,* 91–104.

Imel, Z. E., Baer, J. S., Martino, S., Ball, S. A., & Carroll, K. M. (2011). Mutual influence in therapist competence and adherence to motivational enhancement therapy. *Drug and Alcohol Dependence, 115*(3), 229–236.

Imel, Z. E., Sheng, E., Baldwin, S. A., & Atkins, D. C. (2015). Removing very low-performing therapists: A simulation of performance-based retention in psychotherapy. *Psychotherapy, 52*(3), 329–336.

Imel, Z. E., & Wampold, B. (2008). The importance of treatment and the science of common factors in psychotherapy. In S. D. Brown & R. W. Lent (Eds.), *Handbook of counseling psychology* (pp. 249–266). New York: Wiley.

Imel, Z. E., Wampold, B. E., Miller, S. D., & Fleming, R. R. (2008). Distinctions without a difference: Direct comparisons of psychotherapies for alcohol use disorders. *Psychology of Addictive Behaviors, 22*(4), 533–543.

James, W. (1994/1902). *The varieties of religious experience.* New York: Modern Library Edition.

Janis, I. L. (1959). Decisional conflicts: A theoretical analysis. *Conflict Resolution, 3,* 6–27.

Janis, I. L., & Mann, L. (1976). Coping with decisional conflict. *American Scientist, 64,* 657–666.

Janis, I. L., & Mann, L. (1977). *Decision making: A psychological analysis of conflict, choice and commitment.* New York: Free Press.

Johnson, S. M., & Greenberg, L. S. (1988). Relating process to outcome in marital therapy. *Journal of Marital and Family Therapy, 14*(2), 175–183.

Jones, R. A. (1981). *Self-fulfilling prophecies: Social, psychological, and physiological effects of expectancies.* New York: Psychology Press.

Jung, C. G. (1957). *The undiscovered self: The dilemma of the individual in modern society*. New York: Little, Brown & Company.

Jung, C. G., Read, H., Adler, G., & Hully, R. F. C. (Eds.). (1969). *Collected works of C. G. Jung: Vol. 11. Psychology and religion: West and East* (2nd ed.). Princeton, NJ: Princeton University Press.

Kabat-Zinn, J. (2013). *Full catastrophe living: Using the wisdom of your body and mind to face stress, pain, and illness* (rev. ed.). New York: Bantam Books.

Kabat-Zinn, J. (2016). *Mindfulness for beginners: Reclaiming the present moment— and your life*. Boulder, CO: Sounds True.

Kadden, R. M., Litt, M. D., & Cooney, N. L. (1992). Relationship between role-play measures of coping skills and alcoholism treatment outcomes. *Addictive Behaviors, 17*, 425–437.

Kaptchuk, T. J., Kelley, J. M., Conboy, L. A., Davis, R. B., Kerr, C. E., Jacobson, E. E., . . . Lembo, A. J. (2008). Components of placebo effect: Randomised controlled trial in patients with irritable bowel syndrome. *British Medical Journal, 336*(7651), 999–1003.

Karno, M. P., & Longabaugh, R. (2005). An examination of how therapist directiveness interacts with patient anger and reactance to predict alcohol use. *Journal of Studies on Alcohol, 66*, 825–832.

Karpiak, C. P., & Benjamin, L. S. (2004). Therapist affirmation and the process and outcome of psychotherapy: Two sequential analytic studies. *Journal of Clinical Psychology, 60*(6), 656–659.

Katz, A. D., & Hoyt, W. T. (2014). The influence of multicultural counseling competence and anti-black prejudice on therapists' outcome expectancies. *Journal of Counseling Psychology, 61*(2), 299–305.

Kelley, F. A., Gelso, C. J., Fuertes, J. N., Marmarosh, C., & Lanier, S. H. (2010). The real relationship inventory: Development and psychometric investigation of the client form. *Psychotherapy: Theory, Research, and Practice, 47*(4), 540–553.

Kelm, Z., Womer, J., Walter, J. K., & Feudtner, C. (2014). Interventions to cultivate physician empathy: A systematic review. *BMC Medical Education, 14*(219).

Keng, S.-L., Smoski, M. J., & Robins, C. J. (2011). Effects of mindfulness on psychological health: A review of empirical studies. *Clinical Psychology Review, 31*(6), 1041–1056.

Kiesler, D. J. (1971). Patient experiencing and successful outcome in individual psychotherapy of schizophrenics and psychoneurotics. *Journal of Consulting and Clinical Psychology, 37*(3), 370–385.

Kiesler, D. J., Klein, M. H., Mathieu, P. L., & Schoeninger, D. (1967). Constructive personality change for therapy and control patients. In C. R. Rogers, E. T. Gendlin, D. J. Kiesler, & C. B. Truax (Eds.), *The therapeutic relationship and its impact* (pp. 251–294). Madison: University of Wisconsin Press.

Kiken, L. G., Garland, E. L., Bluth, K., Palsson, O. S., & Gaylord, S. A. (2015). From a state to a trait: Trajectories of state mindfulness in meditation during intervention predict changes in trait mindfulness. *Personality and Individual Differences, 81*, 41–46.

Kim, D.-M., Wampold, B. E., & Bolt, D. M. (2006). Therapist effects in psychotherapy: A random-effects modeling of the National Institute of Mental Health Treatment of Depression Collaborative Research Program data. *Psychotherapy Research, 16*(2), 161–172.

Kirschenbaum, H. (2009). *The life and work of Carl Rogers*. Alexandria, VA: American Counseling Association.

Kirschenbaum, H., & Henderson, V. L. (Eds.). (1989). *Carl Rogers: Dialogues*. Boston: Houghton-Mifflin.

Kivlighan, D. M., Jr., & Holmes, S. E. (2004). The importance of therapeutic factors: A typology of therapeutic factors studies. In J. L. DeLucia-Waack, D. A. Gerrity, C. R. Calodner, & M. T. RIva (Eds.), *Handbook of group counseling and psychotherapy* (pp. 23–36). Thousand Oaks, CA: SAGE.

Klein, M. H., Mathieu-Coughlan, P., & Kiesler, D. J. (1986). The experiencing scales. In L. S. Greenberg & W. M. Pinsof (Eds.), *The psychotherapeutic process: A research handbook* (pp. 21–71). New York: Guilford Press.

Klein, W. M. P., & Harris, P. R. (2010). Self-affirmation enhances attentional bias toward threatening components of a persuasive message. *Psychological Science, 20*(12), 1463–1467.

Klonek, F. E., Lehmann-Willenbrock, N., & Kauffeld, S. (2014). Dynamics of resistance to change: A sequential analysis of change agents in action. *Journal of Change Management, 14*(3), 334–360.

Kluckhohn, C., & Murray, H. A. (Eds.). (1953). *Personality in nature, society, and culture*. New York: Knopf.

Knox, S., & Hill, C. E. (2003). Therapist self-disclosure: Research-based suggestions for practitioners. *Journal of Clinical Psychology, 59*(5), 529–539.

Kobak, K. A., Craske, M. G., Rose, R. D., & Wolitsky-Taylor, K. (2013). Web-based therapist training on cognitive behavior therapy for anxiety disorders: A pilot study. *Psychotherapy, 50*(2), 235–247.

Kohlenberg, B. S., Yeater, E. A., & Kohlenberg, R. J. (1998). Functional analytic psychotherapy, the therapeutic alliance, and brief psychotherapy. In J. D. Safran & J. C. Muran (Eds.), *The therapeutic alliance in brief psychotherapy* (pp. 63–93). Washington, DC: American Psychological Association.

Kohlenberg, R. J., & Tsai, A. G. (1994). Functional analytic psychotherapy: A radical behavioral approach to treatment and integration. *Journal of Psychotherapy Integration, 4*, 175–201.

Kohlenberg, R. J., & Tsai, M. (2007). *Functional analytic psychotherapy: Creating intense and curative therapeutic relationships*. New York: Springer.

Kolden, G. G., Klein, M. H., Wang, C.-C., & Austin, S. B. (2011). Congruence/genuineness. *Psychotherapy, 48*(1), 65–71.

Kolden, G. G., Wang, C.-C., Austin, S. B., Chang, Y., & Klein, M. H. (2018). Congruence/genuineness: A meta-analysis. *Psychotherapy, 55*(4), 424–433.

Koocher, G. P., & Keith-Spiegel, P. (2016). *Ethics in psychology and the mental health professions: Standards and cases* (4th ed.). New York: Oxford University Press.

Kortlever, J. T. P., Ottenhoff, J. S. E., Vagner, G. A., Ring, D., & Reichel, L. M. (2019). Visit duration does not correlate with perceived physician empathy. *Journal of Bone and Joint Surgery, 101*, 296–301.

Kraus, D. R., Bentley, J. H., Alexander, P. C., Boswell, J. F., Constantino, M. J., Baxter, E. E., & Castonguay, L. G. (2016). Predicting therapist effectiveness from their own practice-based evidence. *Journal of Consulting and Clinical Psychology, 84*(6), 473–483.

Krigel, S. W., Grobe, J. E., Goggin, K., Harris, K. J., Moreno, J. L., & Catley, D. (2017). Motivational interviewing and the decisional balance procedure for cessation induction in smokers not intending to quit. *Addictive Behaviors, 64*, 171–178.

Kugelmass, H. (2016). "Sorry, I'm not accepting new patients": An audit study of access to mental health care. *Journal of Health and Social Behavior, 57*(2), 168–183.

Lafferty, P., Beutler, L. E., & Crago, M. (1989). Differences between more and less effective psychotherapists: A study of select therapist variables. *Journal of Consulting and Clinical Psychology, 57*(1), 76–80.

Lamm, C., Batson, C. D., & Decety, J. (2007). The neural substrate of human empathy: Effects of perspective-taking and cognitive appraisal. *Journal of Cognitive Neuroscience, 19*(1), 42–58.

Lane, C., Huws-Thomas, M., Hood, K., Rollnick, S., Edwards, K., & Robling, M. (2005). Measuring adaptations of motivational interviewing: The development and validation of the behavior change counseling index (BECCI). *Patient Education and Counseling, 56*(2), 166–173.

Larson, D. G. (2020). *The helper's journey: Empathy, compassion and the challenge of caring* (2nd ed.). Champaign, IL: Research Press.

Larson, D. G., Chastain, R. L., Hoyt, W. T., & Ayzenberg, R. (2015). Self-concealment: Integrative review and working model. *Journal of Social and Clinical Psychology, 34*(8), 705–774.

Laska, K. M., Gurman, A. S., & Wampold, B. E. (2014). Expanding the lens of evidence-based practice in psychotherapy: A common factors perspective. *Psychotherapy, 51*(4), 467–481.

Lazarus, G., Atzil-Slonim, D., Bar-Kalifa, E., Hasson-Ohayon, I., & Rafaeli, E. (2019). Clients' emotional instability and therapists' inferential flexibility predict therapists' session-by-session empathic accuracy. *Journal of Counseling Psychology, 66*(1), 56–69.

Leake, G. J., & King, A. S. (1977). Effect of counselor expectations on alcoholic recovery. *Alcohol Health and Research World, 1*(3), 16–22.

Lenz, A. S., Rosenbaum, L., & Sheperis, D. (2016). Meta-analysis of randomized controlled trials of motivational enhancement therapy for reducing substance use. *Journal of Addictions and Offender Counseling, 37*(2), 66–86.

Levenson, R. W., & Ruef, A. M. (1992). Empathy: A physiological substrate. *Journal of Personality and Social Psychology, 63*(2), 234–246.

Levitt, H. M., Minami, T., Greenspan, S. B., Puckett, J. A., Henretty, J. R., Reich, C. M., & Berman, J. M. (2016). How therapist self-disclosure relates to alliance and outcomes: A naturalistic study. *Counselling Psychology Quarterly, 29*(1), 7–28.

Levitt, H. M., & Pomerville, A. (2016). A qualitative meta-analysis examining clients' experiences of psychotherapy: A new agenda. *Psychological Bulletin, 142*(8), 801–830.

Lewis, C. S. (1960). *The four loves.* New York: Harcourt Brace.

Lietaer, G. (2001a). Authenticity, congruence and transparency. In D. Brazier (Ed.), *Beyond Carl Rogers: Towards a psychotherapy for the 21st century* (pp. 17–46). London: Constable & Robinson.

Lietaer, G. (2001b). Being genuine as a clinician: Congruence and transparency. In G. Wyatt (Ed.), *Rogers' therapeutic conditions: Evolution, theory and practice: Vol. 1. Congruence* (pp. 36—54). Ross-on-Wye, UK: PCCS Books.

Linehan, M. M. (2014). *DBT skills training manual.* New York: Guilford Press.

Linehan, M. M., Dimeff, L. A., Reynolds, S. K., Comtois, K. A., Welch, S. S., Heagerty, P., & Kivlahan, D. R. (2002). Dialectical behavior therapy versus comprehensive validation therapy plus 12-step for the treatment of opioid dependent women meeting criteria for borderline personality disorder. *Drug and Alcohol Dependence, 67*(1), 13–26.

Litten, R. Z., & Allen, J. P. (1992). *Measuring alcohol consumption: Psychosocial and biochemical methods*. Totowa, NJ: Humana Press.

Locke, E. A., & Latham, G. P. (1990). *A theory of goal setting and task performance*. Englewood Cliffs, NJ: Prentice-Hall.

Longabaugh, R., & Magill, M. (2011). Recent advances in behavioral addiction treatments: Focusing on mechanisms of change. *Current Psychiatry Reports, 13*(5), 383–389.

Longabaugh, R., Magill, M., Morgenstern, J., & Huebner, R. (2013). Mechanisms of behavior change in treatment for alcohol and other drug use disorders. In B. M. McCrady & E. E. Epstein (Eds.), *Addictions: A comprehensive guidebook* (2nd ed., pp. 572–596). New York: Oxford University Press.

Longabaugh, R., Mattson, M. E., Connors, G. J., & Cooney, N. L. (1994). Quality of life as an outcome variable in alcoholism treatment research. *Journal of Studies on Alcohol, 12*(Suppl.), 119–129.

Longabaugh, R., & Wirtz, P. W. (Eds.). (2001). *Project MATCH hypotheses: Results and causal chain analyses* (Project MATCH Monograph Series, Vol. 8). Bethesda, MD: National Institute on Alcohol Abuse and Alcoholism.

Longabaugh, R., Zweben, A., LoCastro, J. S., & Miller, W. R. (2005). Origins, issues and options in the development of the Combined Behavioral Intervention. *Journal of Studies on Alcohol, 66*(4), S179–S187.

Love, P. K., Kilmer, E. D., & Callahan, J. L. (2016). Deliberate interleaving practice in psychotherapy training. *Psychotherapy Bulletin, 51*(2), 16–21.

Luborsky, L., Auerbach, A. H., Chandler, M., Cohen, J., & Bachrach, H. M. (1971). Factors influencing the outcome of psychotherapy: A review of quantitative research. *Psychological Bulletin, 75*(3), 145–185.

Luborsky, L., McLellan, A. T., Diguer, L., Woody, G., & Seligman, D. A. (1997). The psychotherapist matters: Comparison of outcomes across twenty-two therapists and seven patient samples. *Clinical Psychology: Science and Practice, 4*, 53–65.

Luborsky, L., McLellan, A. T., Woody, G. E., O'Brien, C. P., & Auerbach, A. (1985). Therapist success and its determinants. *Archives of General Psychiatry, 42*, 602–611.

Lynch, A., Newlands, F., & Forrester, D. (2019). What does empathy sound like in social work communication?: A mixed-methods study of empathy in child protection social work practice. *Child and Family Social Work, 24*(1), 139–147.

Magill, M., Apodaca, T. R., Barnett, N. P., & Monti, P. M. (2010). The route to change: Within-session predictors of change plan completion in a motivational interview. *Journal of Substance Abuse Treatment, 38*(3), 299–305.

Magill, M., Apodaca, T. R., Borsari, B., Gaume, J., Hoadley, A., Gordon, R. E. F., . . . Moyers, T. (2018). A meta-analysis of motivational interviewing process: Technical, relational, and conditional process models of change. *Journal of Consulting and Clinical Psychology, 86*(2), 140–157.

Magill, M., Bernstein, M. H., Hoadley, A., Borsari, B., Apodaca, T. R., Gaume, J., & Tonigan, J. S. (2019). Do what you say and say what you are going to do: A preliminary meta-analysis of client change and sustain talk subtypes in motivational interviewing. *Psychotherapy Research, 29*(7), 860–869.

Magill, M., Gaume, J., Apodaca, T. R., Walthers, J., Mastroleo, N. R., Borsari, B., & Longabaugh, R. (2014). The technical hypothesis of motivational interviewing: A meta-analysis of MI's key causal model. *Journal of Consulting and Clinical Psychology, 82*(6), 973–983.

Magill, M., & Hallgren, K. A. (2019). Mechanisms of behavior change in motivational interviewing: Do we understand how MI works? *Current Opinion in Psychology, 30,* 1–5.

Magill, M., Janssen, T., Mastroleo, N., Hoadley, A., Walthers, J., Barnett, N., & Colby, S. (2019). Motivational interviewing technical process and moderated relational process with underage young adult heavy drinkers. *Psychology of Addictive Behaviors, 33*(2), 128–138.

Magill, M., Kiluk, B. D., McCrady, B. S., Tonigan, J. S., & Longabaugh, R. (2015). Active ingredients of treatment and client mechanisms of change in behavioral treatments for alcohol use disorders: Progress 10 years later. *Alcoholism: Clinical and Experimental Research, 39*(10), 1852–1862.

Magill, N., Knight, R., McCrone, P., Ismail, K., & Landau, S. (2019). A scoping review of the problems and solutions associated with contamination in trials of complex interventions in mental health. *BMC Medical Research Methodology, 19*(4).

Marker, I., Salvaris, C. A., Thompson, E. M., Tolliday, T., & Norton, P. J. (2019). Client motivation and engagement in transdiagnostic group cognitive behavioral therapy for anxiety disorders: Predictors and outcomes. *Cognitive Therapy and Research, 43*(5), 819–833.

Marshall, C., & Nielsen, A. S. (2020). *Motivatoinal interviewing for leaders in the helping professions: Facilitating change in organizations.* New York: Guilford Press.

Martell, C. R., Dimidjian, S., & Herman-Dunn, R. (2013). *Behavioral activation for depression: A clinician's guide.* New York: Guilford Press.

Martin, M. (1990). On the induction of mood. *Clinical Psychology Review, 10*(6), 669–697.

Martin, P. J., Moore, R. E., & Sterne, A. L. (1977). Therapists as prophets: Their expectancies and treatment outcomes. *Psychotherapy: Theory, Research and Practice, 14*(2), 188–195.

Martin, P. J., Sterne, A. L., Moore, J. E., & Friedmeyer, M. H. (1976). Patient's and therapists' expectancies and treatment outcome: An elusive relationship reexamined. *Research Communications in Psychology, Psychiatry and Behavior, 1*(2), 301–314.

Martin, T., Christopher, P. J., Houck, J. M., & Moyers, T. B. (2011). The structure of client language and drinking outcomes in Project MATCH. *Psychology of Addictive Behaviors, 25*(3), 439–445.

Martino, D., Ball, S. A., Nich, C., Frankforter, T. C., & Carroll, K. M. (2009). Informal discussions in substance abuse treatment sessions. *Journal of Substance Abuse Treatment, 36,* 366–375.

McCambridge, J., Day, M., Thomas, B. A., & Strang, J. (2011). Fidelity to motivational interviewing and subsequent cannabis cessation among adolescents. *Addictive Behaviors, 36,* 749–754.

McClintock, A. S., Anderson, T. M., Patterson, C. L., & Wing, E. H. (2018). Early psychotherapeutic empathy, alliance, and client outcome: Preliminary evidence of indirect effects. *Journal of Clinical Psychology, 74,* 839–848.

McGregor, D. (2006). *The human side of enterprise* (annotated ed.). New York: McGraw Hill.

McHugh, R. K., & Barlow, D. H. (2010). The dissemination and implementation of evidence-based psychological treatments: A review of current efforts. *American Psychologist, 65*(2), 73–84.

McLellan, A. T., Woody, G. E., Luborsky, L., & Goehl, L. (1988). Is the counselor an "active ingredient" in substance abuse rehabilitation?: An examination of treatment success among four counselors. *Journal of Nervous and Mental Disease, 176,* 423–430.

McLeod, B. D. (2009). Understanding why therapy allegiance is linked to clinical outcomes. *Clinical Psychology: Science and Practice, 16*(1), 69–72.

McLeod, B. D., & Weisz, J. R. (2005). The therapy process observational coding system-alliance scale: Measure characteristics and prediction of outcome in usual clinical practice. *Journal of Consulting and Clinical Psychology, 73*(2), 323–333.

McNaughton, J. L. (2009). Brief interventions for depression in primary care: A systematic review. *Canadian Family Physician, 55*(8), 789–796.

McQueen, J., Howe, T. E., Allan, L., Mains, D., & Hardy, V. (2011). Brief interventions for heavy alcohol users admitted to general hospital wards. *Cochrane Database of Systematic Reviews, 10*(8).

Mento, A. J., Steel, R. P., & Karren, R. J. (1987). A meta-analytic study of the effects of goal setting on task performance: 1966–1984. *Organizational Behavior and Human Decision Processes, 39*(1), 52–83.

Messina, I., Palmieri, A., Sambin, M., Kleinbub, J. R., Voci, A., & Calvo, V. (2013). Somatic underpinnings of perceived empathy: The importance of psychotherapy training. *Psychotherapy Research, 23*(2), 169–177.

Miller, S. D., Hubble, M. A., & Chow, D. (2017). Professional development. In T. Rousmaniere, R. K. Goodyear, S. D. Miller, & B. E. Wampold (Eds.), *The cycle of excellence: Using deliberate practice to improve supervision and training* (pp. 23–47). Hoboken, NJ: Wiley.

Miller, S. D., Hubble, M. A., & Chow, D. (2020). *Better results: Using deliberate practice to improve therapeutic effectiveness.* Washington, DC: American Psychological Association.

Miller, W. R. (1978). Behavioral treatment of problem drinkers: A comparative outcome study of three controlled drinking therapies. *Journal of Consulting and Clinical Psychology, 46,* 74–86.

Miller, W. R. (1980). Maintenance of therapeutic change: A usable evaluation design. *Professional Psychology, 11,* 660–663.

Miller, W. R. (1983). Motivational interviewing with problem drinkers. *Behavioural Psychotherapy, 11,* 147–172.

Miller, W. R. (1994). Motivational interviewing: III. On the ethics of motivational intervention. *Behavioural and Cognitive Psychotherapy, 22,* 111–123.

Miller, W. R. (Ed.). (1999). *Integrating spirituality into treatment: Resources for practitioners.* Washington, DC: American Psychological Association.

Miller, W. R. (2000). Rediscovering fire: Small interventions, large effects. *Psychology of Addictive Behaviors, 14,* 6–18.

Miller, W. R. (Ed.). (2004). *Combined Behavioral Intervention manual: A clinical research guide for therapists treating people with alcohol abuse and dependence* (Vol. 1). Bethesda, MD: National Institute on Alcohol Abuse and Alcoholism.

Miller, W. R. (2005). What is human nature?: Reflections from Judeo-Christian perspectives. In W. R. Miller & H. D. Delaney (Eds.), *Judeo-Christian perspectives on psychology: Human nature, motivation, and change* (pp. 11–29). Washington, DC: American Psychological Association.

Miller, W. R. (2015). No more waiting lists! *Substance Use and Misuse, 50*(8–9), 1169–1170.

Miller, W. R. (2017). *Lovingkindness: Realizing and practicing your true self.* Eugene, OR: Wipf & Stock.

Miller, W. R. (2018). *Listening well: The art of empathic understanding*. Eugene, OR: Wipf & Stock.

Miller, W. R., & Baca, L. M. (1983). Two-year follow-up of bibliotherapy and therapist-directed controlled drinking training for problem drinkers. *Behavior Therapy, 14,* 441–448.

Miller, W. R., Benefield, R. G., & Tonigan, J. S. (1993). Enhancing motivation for change in problem drinking: A controlled comparison of two therapist styles. *Journal of Consulting and Clinical Psychology, 61,* 455–461.

Miller, W. R., & C'de Baca, J. (1994). Quantum change: Toward a psychology of transformation. In T. Heatherton & J. Weinberger (Eds.), *Can personality change?* (pp. 253–280). Washington, DC: American Psychological Association.

Miller, W. R., & C'de Baca, J. (2001). *Quantum change: When epiphanies and sudden insights transform ordinary lives*. New York: Guilford Press.

Miller, W. R., & Danaher, B. G. (1976). Maintenance in parent training. In J. D. Krumboltz & C. E. Thoresen (Eds.), *Counseling methods* (pp. 434–444). New York: Holt, Rinehart & Winston.

Miller, W. R., & DiPilato, M. (1983). Treatment of nightmares via relaxation and desensitization: A controlled evaluation. *Journal of Consulting and Clinical Psychology, 51*(6), 870–877.

Miller, W. R., Forcehimes, A. A., & Zweben, A. (2019). *Treating addiction: A guide for professionals* (2nd ed.). New York: Guilford Press.

Miller, W. R., Gribskov, C. J., & Mortell, R. L. (1981). Effectiveness of a self-control manual for problem drinkers with and without therapist contact. *International Journal of the Addictions, 16,* 1247–1254.

Miller, W. R., Hedrick, K. E., & Orlofsky, D. (1991). The Helpful Responses Questionnaire: A procedure for measuring therapeutic empathy. *Journal of Clinical Psychology, 47,* 444–448.

Miller, W. R., LoCastro, J. S., Longabaugh, R., O'Malley, S., & Zweben, A. (2005). When worlds collide: Blending the divergent traditions of pharmacotherapy and psychotherapy outcome research. *Journal of Studies on Alcohol*(Suppl. 15), 17–23.

Miller, W. R., & Meyers, R. J. (1995, Spring). Beyond generic criteria: Reflections on life after clinical science wins. *Clinical Science* (Spring), 4–6.

Miller, W. R., Meyers, R. J., & Tonigan, J. S. (2001). A comparison of CRA and traditional approaches. In R. J. Meyers & W. R. Miller (Eds.), *A community reinforcement approach to addiction treatment* (pp. 62–78). Cambridge, UK: Cambridge University Press.

Miller, W. R., & Mount, K. A. (2001). A small study of training in motivational interviewing: Does one workshop change clinician and client behavior? *Behavioural and Cognitive Psychotherapy, 29,* 457–471.

Miller, W. R., & Moyers, T. B. (2015). The forest and the trees: Relational and specific factors in addiction treatment. *Addiction, 110*(3), 401–413.

Miller, W. R., & Moyers, T. B. (2017). Motivational interviewing and the clinical science of Carl Rogers. *Journal of Consulting and Clinical Psychology, 85*(8), 757–766.

Miller, W. R., Moyers, T. B., Arciniega, L., Ernst, D., & Forcehimes, A. (2005). Training, supervision and quality monitoring of the COMBINE Study behavioral interventions. *Journal of Studies on Alcohol*(Suppl. 15), 188–195.

Miller, W. R., & Muñoz, R. F. (1976). *How to control your drinking*. Englewood Cliffs, NJ: Prentice-Hall.

Miller, W. R., & Rollnick, S. (1991). *Motivational interviewing: Preparing people to change addictive behavior.* New York: Guilford Press.

Miller, W. R., & Rollnick, S. (2004). Talking oneself into change: Motivational interviewing, stages of change, and the therapeutic process. *Journal of Cognitive Psychotherapy, 18,* 299–308.

Miller, W. R., & Rollnick, S. (2013). *Motivational interviewing: Helping people change* (3rd ed.). New York: Guilford Press.

Miller, W. R., & Rollnick, S. (2014). The effectiveness and ineffectiveness of complex behavioral interventions: Impact of treatment fidelity. *Contemporary Clinical Trials, 37*(2), 234–241.

Miller, W. R., Rollnick, S., & Moyers, T. B. (2013). *Motivational interviewing: Helping people change* [DVD series]. Carson City, NV: Change Companies.

Miller, W. R., & Rose, G. S. (2009). Toward a theory of motivational interviewing. *American Psychologist, 64*(6), 527–537.

Miller, W. R., & Rose, G. S. (2010). Motivational interviewing in relational context. *American Psychologist, 65*(4), 298–299.

Miller, W. R., & Rose, G. S. (2015). Motivational interviewing and decisional balance: Contrasting responses to client ambivalence. *Behavioural and Cognitive Psychotherapy, 43*(2), 129–141.

Miller, W. R., & Sanchez, V. C. (1994). Motivating young adults for treatment and lifestyle change. In G. Howard (Ed.), *Issues in alcohol use and misuse by young adults* (pp. 55–82). Notre Dame, IN: University of Notre Dame Press.

Miller, W. R., Sorensen, J. L., Selzer, J. A., & Brigham, G. S. (2006). Disseminating evidence-based practices in substance abuse treatment: A review with suggestions. *Journal of Substance Abuse Treatment, 31*(1), 25–39.

Miller, W. R., Taylor, C. A., & West, J. (1980). Focused versus broad-spectrum behavior therapy for problem drinkers. *Journal of Consulting and Clinical Psychology, 48*(5), 590–601.

Miller, W. R., Tonigan, J. S., & Longabaugh, R. (1995). *The Drinker Inventory of Consequences (DrInC): An instrument for assessing adverse consequences of alcohol abuse.* Bethesda, MD: National Institute on Alcohol Abuse and Alcoholism.

Miller, W. R., Toscova, R. T., Miller, J. H., & Sanchez, V. (2000). A theory based motivational approach for reducing alcohol/drug problems in college. *Health Education and Behavior, 27,* 744–759.

Miller, W. R., Walters, S. T., & Bennett, M. E. (2001). How effective is alcoholism treatment in the United States? *Journal of Studies on Alcohol, 62,* 211–220.

Miller, W. R., & Wilbourne, P. L. (2002). Mesa Grande: A methodological analysis of clinical trials of treatment for alcohol use disorders. *Addiction, 97*(3), 265–277.

Miller, W. R., Yahne, C. E., Moyers, T. B., Martinez, J., & Pirritano, M. (2004). A randomized trial of methods to help clinicians learn motivational interviewing. *Journal of Consulting and Clinical Psychology, 72*(6), 1050–1062.

Miller, W. R., Yahne, C. E., & Tonigan, J. S. (2003). Motivational interviewing in drug abuse services: A randomized trial. *Journal of Consulting and Clinical Psychology, 71,* 754–763.

Miller, W. R., Zweben, J. E., & Johnson, W. (2005). Evidence-based treatment: Why, what, where, when, and how? *Journal of Substance Abuse Treatment, 29,* 267–276.

Mohr, D. C. (1995). Negative outcome in psychotherapy: A critical review. *Clinical Science and Practice, 2*(1), 1–27.

Monahan, J. (Ed.). (1980). *Who is the client?: The ethics of psychological intervention in the criminal justice system*. Washington, DC: American Psychological Association.

Moos, R. H. (2007). Theory-based processes that promote the remission of substance use disorders. *Clinical Psychology Review, 27*(5), 537–551.

Morche, J., Mathes, T., & Pieper, D. (2016). Relationship between surgeon volume and outcomes: A systematic review of systematic reviews. *Systematic Reviews, 5*(204).

Morgenstern, J., & Longabaugh, R. (2000). Cognitive-behavioral treatment for alcohol dependence: A review of evidence for its hypothesized mechanisms of action. *Addiction, 95*, 1475–1490.

Mowat, A., Maher, C., & Ballard, E. (2016). Surgical outcomes for low-volume vs high-volume surgeons in gynecology surgery: A systematic review and meta-analysis. *American Journal of Obstetrics, 215*(1), 21–33.

Moyer, A., Finney, J. W., Swearingen, C. E., & Vergun, P. (2002). Brief interventions for alcohol problems: A meta-analytic review of controlled investigations in treatment-seeking and non-treatment-seeking populations. *Addiction, 97*(3), 279–292.

Moyers, T. B., Houck, J. M., Glynn, L. H., Hallgren, K. A., & Manual, J. K. (2017). A randomized controlled trial to influence client language in substance use disorder treatment. *Drug and Alcohol Dependence, 172*, 43–50.

Moyers, T. B., Houck, J. M., Rice, S. L., Longabaugh, R., & Miller, W. R. (2016). Therapist empathy, combined behavioral intervention, and alcohol outcomes in the COMBINE research project. *Journal of Consulting and Clinical Psychology, 84*(3), 221–229.

Moyers, T. B., Manuel, J. K., Wilson, P., Hendrickson, S. M. L., Talcott, W., & Durand, P. (2008). A randomized trial investigating training in motivational interviewing for behavioral health providers. *Behavioural and Cognitive Psychotherapy, 36*, 149–162.

Moyers, T. B., & Martin, T. (2006). Therapist influence on client language during motivational interviewing sessions. *Journal of Substance Abuse Treatment, 30*(3), 245–252.

Moyers, T. B., Martin, T., Catley, D., Harris, K. J., & Ahluwalia, J. S. (2003). Assessing the integrity of motivational interventions: Reliability of the Motivational Interviewing Skills Code. *Behavioural and Cognitive Psychotherapy, 31*, 177–184.

Moyers, T. B., Martin, T., Christopher, P. J., Houck, J. M., Tonigan, J. S., & Amrhein, P. C. (2007). Client language as a mediator of motivational interviewing efficacy: Where is the evidence? *Alcoholism: Clinical and Experimental Research, 31*(10, Suppl.), 40s–47s.

Moyers, T. B., Martin, T., Houck, J. M., Christopher, P. J., & Tonigan, J. S. (2009). From in-session behaviors to drinking outcomes: A causal chain for motivational interviewing. *Journal of Consulting and Clinical Psychology, 77*(6), 1113–1124.

Moyers, T. B., Martin, T., Manuel, J. K., Hendrickson, S. M. L., & Miller, W. R. (2005). Assessing competence in the use of motivational interviewing. *Journal of Substance Abuse Treatment, 28*, 19–26.

Moyers, T. B., & Miller, W. R. (2013). Is low therapist empathy toxic? *Psychology of Addictive Behaviors, 27*(3), 878–884.

Moyers, T. B., Miller, W. R., & Hendrickson, S. M. L. (2005). How does motivational interviewing work?: Therapist interpersonal skill predicts client involvement within motivational interviewing sessions. *Journal of Consulting and Clinical Psychology, 73*(4), 590–598.

Moyers, T. B., Rowell, L. N., Manuel, J. K., Ernst, D., & Houck, J. M. (2016). The Motivational Interviewing Treatment Integrity code (MITI 4): Rationale, preliminary reliability and validity. *Journal of Substance Abuse Treatment, 65*, 36–42.

Mulder, R., Murray, G., & Rucklidge, J. (2017). Common versus specific factors in psychotherapy: Opening the black box. *The Lancet Psychiatry, 4*(12), 953–962.

Muran, J. C., Safran, J. D., Eubanks, C. F., & Gorman, B. S. (2018). The effect of alliance-focused training on a cognitive-behavioral therapy for personality disorders. *Journal of Consulting and Clinical Psychology, 86*(4), 384–397.

Najavits, L. M., & Weiss, R. D. (1994). Variations in therapist effectiveness in the treatment of patients with substance use disorders: An empirical review. *Addiction, 89*, 679–688.

Napel-Schutz, M. C., Abma, T. A., Bamelis, L. L. M., & Arntz, A. (2017). How to train experienced therapists in a new method: A qualitative study into therapists' views. *Clinical Psychology and Psychotherapy, 24*(2), 359–372.

Nenkov, G. Y., & Gollwitzer, P. M. (2012). Pre- versus postdecisional deliberation and goal commitment: The positive effects of defensiveness. *Journal of Experimental Social Psychology, 48*, 106–121.

Neubert, M. J. (1998). The value of feedback and goal setting over goal setting alone and potential moderators of this effect: A meta-analysis. *Human Performance, 11*(4), 321–335.

Nichols, M. P. (2009). *The lost art of listening: How learning to listen can improve relationships* (2nd ed.). New York: Guilford Press.

Nock, M. K. (2007). Conceptual and design essentials for evaluating mechanisms of change. *Alcoholism: Clinical and Experimental Research, 31*(10, Suppl.), 4s–12s.

Norcross, J. C. (Ed.). (2011). *Psychotherapy relationships that work: Evidence-based responsiveness* (2nd ed.). New York: Oxford University Press.

Norcross, J. C., & Wampold, B. E. (2011). Evidence-based therapy relationships: Research conclusions and clinical practice. In J. C. Norcross (Ed.), *Psychotherapy relationships that work: Evidence-based responsiveness* (2nd ed., pp. 423–430). New York: Oxford University Press.

Norcross, J. C., & Wampold, B. E. (2019). Evidence-based psychotherapy responsiveness: The third task force. In J. C. Norcross & B. E. Wampold (Eds.), *Psychotherapy relationships that work: Vol. 2. Evidence-based therapist responsiveness* (3rd ed., pp. 1–14). New York: Oxford University Press.

Norris, L. A., Rifkin, L. S., Olino, T. M., Piacenti, J., Albano, A. M., Birmaher, B., . . . Kendall, P. C. (2019). Multi-informant expectancies and treatment outcomes for anxiety in youth. *Child Psychiatry and Human Development, 50*, 1002–1010.

Norton, P. J., & Little, T. E. (2014). Does experience matter?: Trainee experience and outcomes during transdiagnostic cognitive-behavioral group therapy for anxiety. *Cognitive Behaviour Therapy, 43*(3), 230–238.

Nuro, K. F., Maccarelli, L., Baker, S. M., Martino, S., Rounsaville, B. J., & Carroll, K. M. (2005). *Yale Adherence and Competence Scale (YACS II) guidelines* (2nd ed.). New Haven, CT: Yale University.

O'Halloran, P. D., Shields, N., Blackstock, F., Wintle, E., & Taylor, N. F. (2016). Motivational interviewing increases physical activity and self-efficacy in people living in the community after hip fracture: A randomized controlled trial. *Clinical Rehabilitation, 30*(11), 1108–1119.

Okamoto, A., Dattilio, F. M., Dobson, K. S., & Kazantzis, N. (2019). The therapeutic relationship in cognitive-behavioral therapy: Essential features and common challenges. *Practice Innovations, 4*(2), 112–123.

Okiishi, J., Lambert, M. J., Nielsen, S. L., & Ogles, B. M. (2003). Waiting for supershrink: An empirical analysis of therapist effects. *Clinical Psychology and Psychotherapy, 10,* 361–373.

Orlinsky, D. E., Grawe, K., & Parks, B. K. (1994). Process and outcome in psychotherapy: Noch einmal. In A. E. Bergin & S. L. Garfield (Eds.), *Handbook of psychotherapy and behavior change* (pp. 270–376). New York: Wiley.

Orlinsky, D. E., & Howard, K. I. (1986). Process and outcome in psychotherapy. In S. L. Garfield & A. E. Bergin (Eds.), *Handbook of psychotherapy and behavior change* (3rd ed., pp. 311–381). New York: Wiley.

Ottman, K., Kohrt, B. A., Pedersen, G., & Schafer, A. (2020). Use of role plays to assess therapist competency and its association with client outcomes in psychological interventions: A scoping review and competency research agenda. *Behaviour Research and Therapy, 130*(103531).

Owen, J., Drinane, J. M., Kivlighan, M., Miller, S., Kopta, M., & Imel, Z. (2019). Are high-performing therapists both effective and consistent? A test of therapist expertise. *Journal of Consulting and Clinical Psychology, 87*(12), 1149–1156.

Owen, J., Miller, S. D., Seidel, J., & Chow, D. (2016). The working alliance in treatment of military adolescents. *Journal of Consulting and Clinical Psychology, 84*(3), 200–210.

Pascuel-Leone, A., & Yervomenko, N. (2017). The client "experiencing" scale as a predictor of treatment outcomes: A meta-analysis on psychotherapy process. *Psychotherapy Research, 27*(6), 653–665.

Patterson, G. R., & Chamberlain, P. (1994). A functional analysis of resistance during patient training therapy. *Clinical Psychology: Science and Practice, 1*(1), 53–70.

Patterson, G. R., & Forgatch, M. S. (1985). Therapist behavior as a determinant for client noncompliance: A paradox for the behavior modifier. *Journal of Consulting and Clinical Psychology, 53*(6), 846–851.

Perez-Rosas, V., Wu, X., Resnicow, K., & Mihalcea, R. (2019). What makes a good counselor?: Learning to distinguish between high-quality and low-quality counseling conversations. In P. Nakov & A. Palmer, *Proceedings of the 57th annual meeting of the Association for Computational Linguistics* (pp. 926–935), Florence, Italy.

Peterson, C., & Seligman, M. E. P. (2004). *Character strengths and virtues: A handbook and classification.* New York: Oxford University Press.

Pfeiffer, E., Ormhaug, S., Tutus, D., Holt, T., Rosner, R., Larsen, T., & Jensen, T. (2020). Does the therapist matter?: Therapist characteristics and their relation to outcome in trauma-focused cognitive behavioral therapy for children and adolescents. *European Journal of Psychotraumatology, 11*(1), 1776048.

Pierson, H. M., Hayes, S. C., Gifford, E. V., Roget, N., Padilla, M., Bissett, R., . . . Fisher, G. (2007). An examination of the Motivational Interviewing Treatment Integrity code. *Journal of Substance Abuse Treatment, 32,* 11–17.

Pieterse, A. L., Lee, M., Ritmeester, A., & Collins, N. M. (2013). Towards a model of self-awareness development for counselling and psychotherapy training. *Counseling Psychology Quarterly, 26*(2), 190–207.

Pope, K. S., & Tabachnick, B. G. (1993). Therapists' anger, hate, fear, and sexual feelings: National survey of therapist responses, client characteristics, critical events, formal complaints, and training. *Professional Psychology: Research and Practice, 24*(2), 142–152.

Prestwich, A., Kellar, I., Parker, R., MacRae, S., Learmonth, M., Sykes, B., . . . Castle, H. (2014). How can self-efficacy be increased? Meta-analysis of dietary interventions. *Health Psychology Review, 8*(3), 270–285.

Prochaska, J. O. (1994). Strong and weak principles for progressing from precontemplation to action on the basis of twelve problem behaviors. *Health Psychology, 13,* 47–51.

Prochaska, J. O., & DiClemente, C. C. (1984). *The transtheoretical approach: Crossing traditional boundaries of therapy.* Homewood, IL: Dow/Jones Irwin.

Prochaska, J. O., & Velicer, W. F. (1997). The transtheoretical model of health behavior change. *American Journal of Health Promotion, 12*(1), 38–48.

Prochaska, J. O., Velicer, W. F., Rossi, J. S., Goldstein, M. G., Marcus, B. H., Rakowski, W., . . . Rossi, S. R. (1994). Stages of change and decisional balance for 12 problem behaviors. *Health Psychology, 13*(1), 39–46.

Project MATCH Research Group. (1997). Matching alcoholism treatments to client heterogeneity: Project MATCH posttreatment drinking outcomes. *Journal of Studies on Alcohol, 58*(1), 7–29.

Project MATCH Research Group. (1998). Therapist effects in three treatments for alcohol problems. *Psychotherapy Research, 8,* 455–474.

Raingruber, B. (2003). Video-cued narrative reflection: A research approach for articulating tacit, relational, and embodied understandings. *Qualitative Health Research, 13*(8), 1155–1169.

Rains, S. A. (2013). The nature of psychological reactance revisited: A meta-analytic review. *Human Communication Research, 39*(1), 47–73.

Rakel, D. (2018). *The compassionate connection: The healing power of empathy and mindful listening.* New York: Norton.

Rakovshik, S. G., McManus, F., Vazquez-Montes, M., Muse, K., & Ougrin, D. (2016). Is supervision necessary?: Examining the effects of Internet-based CBT training with and without supervision. *Journal of Consulting and Clinical Psychology, 84*(3), 191–199.

Rashid, T., & Seligman, M. P. (2018). *Positive psychotherapy: Clinician manual.* New York: Oxford University Press.

Richards, S. P., & Bergin, A. E. (1997). *A spiritual strategy for counseling and psychotherapy.* Washington, DC: American Psychological Association.

Robichaud, L. K. (2004). *Depth of experiencing as a client prognostic variable in emotion-focused therapy for adult survivors of childhood abuse.* Master's thesis, University of Windsor, Windsor, Ontario. Retrieved from *https://scholar.uwindsor.ca/cgi/viewcontent.cgi?article=2641&context=etd.*

Rogers, C. R. (1951). *Client-centered therapy.* New York: Houghton Mifflin.

Rogers, C. R. (1957). The necessary and sufficient conditions of therapeutic personality change. *Journal of Consulting Psychology, 21*(2), 95–103.

Rogers, C. R. (1959). A theory of therapy, personality, and interpersonal relationships as developed in the client-centered framework. In S. Koch (Ed.), *Psychology: The study of a science: Vol. 3. Formulations of the person and the social contexts* (pp. 184–256). New York: McGraw-Hill.

Rogers, C. R. (1961). *On becoming a person: A therapist's view of psychotherapy.* Boston: Houghton Mifflin.

Rogers, C. R. (1962). The nature of man. In S. Doniger (Ed.), *The nature of man in theological and psychological perspective* (pp. 91–96). New York: Harper & Brothers.

Rogers, C. R. (1980a). Can learning encompass both ideas and feelings? In *A way of being* (pp. 263–291). New York: Houghton Mifflin.

Rogers, C. R. (1980b). Empathic: An unappreciated way of being. In *A way of being* (pp. 137–163). New York: Houghton Mifflin.

Rogers, C. R. (1980c). The foundations of a person-centered approach. In *A way of being* (pp. 113–136). Boston: Houghton Mifflin.

Rogers, C. R. (1980d). *A way of being.* Boston: Houghton Mifflin.

Rogers, C. R., Gendlin, E. T., Kiesler, D. J., & Truax, C. B. (Eds.). (1967). *The therapeutic relationship and its impact: A study of psychotherapy with schizophrenics.* Westport, CT: Greenwood Press.

Rogers, E. M. (2003). *Diffusion of innovations* (5th ed.). New York: Free Press.

Rohsenow, D. R., & Marlatt, G. A. (1981). The balanced placebo design: Methodological considerations. *Addictive Behaviors, 6,* 107–122.

Rokeach, M. (1973). *The nature of human values.* New York: Free Press.

Rollnick, S., Fader, J. S., Breckon, J., & Moyers, T. B. (2019). *Coaching athletes to be their best: Motivational interviewing in sports.* New York: Guilford Press.

Rollnick, S., Kaplan, S. G., & Rutschman, R. (2016). *Motivational interviewing in schools: Conversations to improve behavior and learning.* New York: Guilford Press.

Rollnick, S., & Miller, W. R. (1995). What is motivational interviewing? *Behavioural and Cognitive Psychotherapy, 23,* 325–334.

Rollnick, S., Miller, W. R., & Butler, C. C. (2008). *Motivational interviewing in health care: Helping patients change behavior.* New York: Guilford Press.

Rollnick, S., Miller, W. R., & Butler, C. C. (in press). *Motivational interviewing in health care* (2nd ed.). New York: Guilford Press.

Rosengren, D. B. (2018). *Building motivational interviewing skills: A practitioner workbook* (2nd ed.). New York: Guilford Press.

Rosenthal, R., & Jacobson, L. (1966). Teachers' expectancies: Determinants of pupils' IQ gains. *Psychological Reports, 19,* 115–118.

Rousmaniere, T., Goodyear, R. K., Miller, S. D., & Wampold, B. E. (2017). *The cycle of excellence: Using deliberate practice to improve supervision and training.* Hoboken, NJ: Wiley.

Rubies-Davis, C. M., & Rosenthal, R. (2016). Intervening in teachers' expectations: A random effects meta-analytic approach to examining the effectiveness of an intervention. *Learning and Individual Differences, 50,* 83–92.

Rubino, G., Barker, C., Roth, T., & Fearon, P. (2000). Therapist empathy and depth of interpretation in response to potential alliance ruptures: The role of therapist and patient attachment styles. *Psychotherapy Research, 10,* 408–420.

Rutter, M. (2006). Implications of resilience concepts for scientific understanding. *Annals of the New York Academy of Sciences, 1094,* 1–12.

Rutter, M. (2013). Annual Research Review: Resilience–Clinical implications. *Journal of Child Psychology and Psychiatry, 54*(4), 474–487.

Ryan, R. M., & Deci, E. L. (2008). A self-determination theory approach to psychotherapy: The motivational basis for effective change. *Candian Psychology, 49,* 186–193.

Ryan, R. M., & Deci, E. L. (2017). *Self-determination theory: Basic psychological needs in motivation, development, and wellness.* New York: Guilford Press.

Sacco, P., Ting, L., Crouch, T. B., Emery, L., Moreland, M., Bright, C., . . . DiClemente, C. (2017). SBIRT training in social work education: Evaluating change using standardized patient simulation. *Journal of Social Work Practice in the Addictions, 17*(1–2), 150–168.

Safran, J. D., Crocker, P., McMain, S., & Murray, P. (1990). Therapeutic alliance rupture as a therapy event for empirical investigation. *Psychotherapy: Theory, Research, Practice, Training, 27*(2), 154–165.

Safran, J. D., & Muran, J. C. (2000). *Negotiating the therapeutic alliance: A relational treatment guide*. New York: Guilford Press.

Safran, J. D., Muran, J. C., Demaria, A., Boutwell, C., Eubanks-Carter, C., & Winston, A. (2014). Investigating the impact of alliance-focused training on interpersonal process and therapists' capacity for experiential reflection. *Psychotherapy Research, 24*(3), 269–285.

Salzberg, S. (1995). *Lovingkindness: The revolutionary art of happiness*. Boston: Shambhala.

Samson, J. E., & Tanner-Smith, E. E. (2015). Single-session alcohol interventions for heavy drinking college students: A systematic review and meta-analysis. *Journal of Studies on Alcohol and Drugs, 76*(4), 530–543.

Sandell, R., Lazar, A., Grant, J., Carlsson, J., Schubert, J., & Broberg, J. (2006). Therapist attitudes and patient outcomes: III. A latent class analysis of therapists. *Psychology and Psychotherapy: Theory, Research and Practice, 79*(4), 629-647.

Schmidt, M. M., & Miller, W. R. (1983). Amount of therapist contact and outcome in a multidimensional depression treatment program. *Acta Psychiatrica Scandinavica, 67*, 319–332.

Schnellbacher, J., & Leijssen, M. (2009). The significance of therapist genuineness from the client's perspective. *Journal of Humanistic Psychology, 49*(2), 207–228.

Schofield, W. (1964). *Psychotherapy: The purchase of friendship*. Englewood Cliffs, NJ: Prentice-Hall.

Schottke, H., Fluckiger, C., Goldberg, S. B., Eversmann, J., & Lange, J. (2017). Predicting psychotherapy outcome based on therapist interpersonal skills: A five-year longitudinal study of a therapist assessment protocol. *Psychotherapy Research: Journal of the Society for Psychotherapy Research, 27*(6), 642–652.

Schumann, A., Meyer, C., Rumpf, H.-J., Hannover, W., Hapke, U., & John, U. (2005). Stage of change transitions and processes of change: Decisional balance and self-efficacy in smokers: A transtheoretical model validation using longitudinal data. *Psychology of Addictive Behaviors, 19*(1), 3–9.

Schwartz, R. A., Chambless, D. L., McCarthy, K. S., Milrod, B., & Barber, J. P. (2019). Client resistance predicts outcomes in cognitive-behavioral therapy for panic disorder. *Psychotherapy Research, 29*(8), 1020–1032.

Seligman, M. E. P. (2012). *Flourish: A visionary new understanding of happiness and well-being*. New York: Free Press.

Shafranske, E. P. (Ed.). (1996). *Religion and the clinical practice of psychology*. Washington, DC: American Psychological Association.

Shapiro, A. K. (1971). Placebo effects in medicine, psychotherapy, and psychoanalysis. In A. E. Bergin & S. L. Garfield (Eds.), *Handbook of psychotherapy and behavior change: An empirical analysis* (pp. 439–473). New York: Wiley.

Shapiro, R. (2006). *The sacred art of lovingkindness: Preparing to practice*. Woodstock, VT: Skylight Paths.

Shapiro, S. L., Astin, J. A., Bishop, S. R., & Cordova, M. (2005). Mindfulness-based stress reduction for health care professionals: Results from a randomized trial. *International Journal of Stress Management, 12*(2), 164–176.

Shaw, B. F. (1999). How to use the allegiance effect to maximize competence and therapeutic outcomes. *Clinical Psychology: Science and Practice, 6*(1), 131–132.

Shaw, C. K., & Shrum, W. F. (1972). The effects of response-contingent reward on the connected speech of children who stutter. *Journal of Speech, Language, and Hearing Research, 37*(1), 75–88.

Sheeran, P., Maki, A., Montanaro, E., Avishai-Yitshak, A., Bryan, A., Klein, W. M. P., . . . Rothman, A. J. (2016). The impact of changing attitudes, norms, and self-efficacy on health-related intentions and behavior: A meta-analysis. *Health Psychology, 35*(11), 1178–1188.

Sherman, D. K. (2013). Self-affirmation: Understanding the effects. *Social and Personality Psychology Compass, 7*(11), 834–845.

Singla, D. R., Hollon, S. D., Velleman, R., Weobong, B., Nadkarni, A., Fairburn, C. G., . . . Patel, V. (2020). Temporal pathways of change in two randomized controlled trials for depression and harmful drinking in Goa, India. *Psychological Medicine, 50*(1), 68–76.

Smedslund, G., Berg, R. C., Hammerstrom, K. T., Steiro, A., Leiknes, K. A., Dahl, H. M., & Karlsen, K. (2011). Motivational interviewing for substance abuse. *Cochrane Database of Systematic Reviews*(5).

Smith, D. D., Kellar, J., Walters, E. L., Reibling, E. T., Phan, T., & Green, S. M. (2016). Does emergency physician empathy reduce thoughts of litigation?: A randomized trial. *Emergency Medicine Journal, 33*, 548–552.

Smith, M. L., Glass, G. V., & Miller, T. I. (1980). *The benefits of psychotherapy.* Baltimore: Johns Hopkins University Press.

Snyder, C. R. (1994). *The psychology of hope.* New York: Free Press.

Snyder, C. R., Ilardi, S. S., Cheavens, H., Michael, S. T., Yamhure, L., & Sympson, S. (2000). The role of hope in cognitive-behavior therapies. *Cognitive Therapy and Research, 24*(6), 747–762.

Snyder, C. R., Michael, S. T., & Cheavens, J. S. (1999). Hope as psychotherapeutic foundation of common factors, placebos, and expectancies. In M. A. Hubble, B. L. Duncan, & S. D. Miller (Eds.), *The heart and soul of change: What works in therapy* (pp. 179–200). Washington, DC: American Psychological Association.

Soma, C. S., Baucom, B. R. W., Xiao, B., Butner, J. E., Hilpert, P., Narayanan, S., . . . Imel, Z. E. (2020). Coregulation of therapist and client emotion during psychotherapy. *Psychotherapy Research, 30*(5), 591–603.

Somers, A. D., Pomerantz, A. M., Meeks, J. T., & Pawlow, L. A. (2014). Should psychotherapists disclose their own psychological problems? *Counselling and Psychotherapy Research, 14*(4), 249–255.

Stack, L. C., Lannon, P. B., & Miley, A. D. (1983). Accuracy of clinicians' expectancies for psychiatric rehospitalization. *American Journal of Community Psychology, 11*(1), 99–113.

Stead, L. F., Buitrago, D., Preciado, N., Sanchez, G., Hartmann-Boyce, J., & Lancaster, T. (2013). Physician advice for smoking cessation. *Cochrane Database of Systematic Reviews, 5*.

Steinberg, M. P., & Miller, W. R. (2015). *Motivational interviewing in diabetes care.* New York: Guilford Press.

Steindl, C., Jonas, E., Sittenthaler, S., Traut-Mattausch, E., & Greenberg, J. (2015). Understanding psychological reactance: New developments and findings. *Zeitschrift für Psychologie, 223*, 205–214.

Stiles, W. B., Honos-Webb, L., & Surko, M. (1998). Responsiveness in psychotherapy. *Clinical Psychology: Science and Practice, 5*(4), 439–458.

Stiles, W. B., McDaniel, S. H., & Gaughey, K. (1979). Verbal response mode correlates of experiencing. *Journal of Consulting and Clinical Psychology, 47*(4), 795–797.

Stinson, J. D., & Clark, M. D. (2017). *Motivational interviewing with offenders: Engagement, rehabilitation, and reentry.* New York: Guilford Press.

Strauss, A. Y., Huppert, J. D., Simpson, H. B., & Foa, E. (2018). What matters more?: Common or specific factors in cognitive-behavioral therapy for OCD: Therapeutic alliance and expectations as predictors of treatment outcome. *Behaviour Research and Therapy, 105,* 43–51.

Strupp, H. H. (1960). *Psychotherpists in action: Explorations of the therapist's contribution to the treatment process.* New York: Grune & Stratton.

Sue, D. W., & Sue, D. (2015). *Counseling the culturally diverse: Theory and practice* (7th ed.). New York: Wiley.

Suzuki, J. Y., & Farber, B. A. (2016). Toward greater specificity of the concept of positive regard. *Person-Centered and Experiential Psychotherapies, 15*(4), 263–284.

Swoboda, C. M., Miller, C. K., & Wills, C. E. (2017). Impact of a goal setting and decision support telephone coaching intervention on diet, psychosocial, and decision outcomes among people with Type 2 diabetes. *Patient Education and Counseling, 100*(7), 1367–1373.

Szumski, G., & Karwowski, M. (2019). Exploring the Pygmalion effect: The role of teacher expectations, academic self-concept, and class context in students' math achievement. *Contemporary Educational Psychology, 59*(101787).

Teasdale, A. C., & Hill, C. E. (2006). Preferences of therapists-in-training for client characteristics. *Psychotherapy: Theory, Research and Practice, 43*(1), 111–118.

Thich Nhat Hanh. (2015). *The miracle of mindfulness: An introduction to the practice of meditation* (Mobi Ho, Trans.). Boston: Beacon Press.

Thwaites, R., Bennett-Levy, J., Cairns, L., Lowrie, R., Robinson, A., Haaroff, B., . . . Perry, H. (2017). Self-practice/self-reflection as a training strategy to enhance therapeutic empathy in low intensity CBT practioners. *New Zealand Journal of Psychology, 46*(2), 63–70.

Tracey, T. J. G., Wampold, B. E., Lichtenberg, J. W., & Goodyear, R. K. (2014). Expertise in psychotherapy: An elusive goal? *American Psychologist, 69*(3), 218–229.

Truax, C. B. (1966). Reinforcement and non-reinforcement in Rogerian psychotherapy. *Journal of Abnormal Psychology, 71,* 1–9.

Truax, C. B., & Carkhuff, R. R. (1965). The experimental manipulation of therapeutic conditions. *Journal of Consulting Psychology, 29,* 119–124.

Truax, C. B., & Carkhuff, R. R. (1967). *Toward effective counseling and psychotherapy.* Chicago: Aldine.

Truax, C. B., & Carkhuff, R. R. (1976). *Toward effective counseling and psychotherapy: Training and practice.* New Brunswick, NJ: Aldine Transaction.

Truijens, F., Zühlke-Van Hulzen, L., & Vanheule, S. (2019). To manualize, or not to manualize: Is that still the question?: A systematic review of empirical evidence for manual superiority in psychological treatment. *Journal of Clinical Psychology, 75,* 329–343.

Tryon, G. S., & Winograd, G. (2011). Goal consensus and collaboration. *Psychotherapy, 48*(1), 50–57.

Tubbs, M. E. (1986). Goal setting: A meta-analytic examination of the empirical evidence. *Journal of Applied Psychology, 71*(3), 474–493.

Turner, J. A., Deyo, R. A., Loeser, J. D., Con Korff, M., & Fordyce, W. E. (1994). The importance of placebo effects in pain treatment and research. *Journal of the American Medical Association, 271,* 1609–1614.

Vader, A. M., Walters, S. T., Prabhu, G. C., Houck, J. M., & Field, C. A. (2010).

The language of motivational interviewing and feedback: Counselor language, client language, and client drinking outcomes. *Psychology of Addictive Behaviors, 24*(2), 190–197.

Valle, S. K. (1981). Interpersonal functioning of alcoholism counselors and treatment outcome. *Journal of Studies on Alcohol, 42,* 783–790.

Vallis, T. M., Shaw, B. F., & Dobson, K. S. (1986). The Cognitive Therapy Scale: Psychometric properties. *Journal of Consulting and Clinical Psychology, 54*(3), 381–385.

van Bentham, P., Spijkerman, R., Blanken, P., Kleinjan, M., Vermeiren, R. J. M., & Hendriks, V. M. (in press). A dual perspective on first-session therapeutic alliance: Strong predictor of youth mental health and addiction treatment outcome. *European Child and Adolescent Psychiatry.*

van Oppen, P., van Balkom, A. J. L. M., Smit, J. H., Schuurmans, J., van Dyck, R., & Emmelkamp, P. M. G. (2010). Does the therapy manual or the therapist matter most in treatment of obsessive-compulsive disorder?: A randomized controlled trial of exposure with response or ritual prevention in 118 patients. *Journal of Clinical Psychiatry, 71*(9), 1158–1167.

Vanier, J. (1998). *Becoming human.* New York: Paulist Press.

Varble, D. L. (1968). Relationship between the therapists' approach-avoidance reactions to hostility and client behavior in therapy. *Journal of Consulting and Clinical Psychology, 32*(3), 237–242.

Vasilaki, E. I., Hosier, S. G., & Cox, W. M. (2006). The efficacy of motivational interviewing as a brief intervention for excessive drinking: A meta-analytic review. *Alcohol and Alcoholism, 41*(3), 328–335.

Vijay, G. C., Wilson, E. C. F., Suhrcke, M., Hardeman, W., Sutton, S., & VBI Programme Team. (2016). Are brief interventions to increase physical activity cost-effective? A systematic review. *British Journal of Sports Medicine, 50,* 408–417.

Villarosa-Hurlocker, M. C., O'Sickey, A. J., Houck, J. M., & Moyers, T. B. (2019). Examining the influence of active ingredients of motivational interviewing on client change talk. *Journal of Substance Abuse Treatment, 96,* 39–45.

Waldron, H. B., Miller, W. R., & Tonigan, J. S. (2001). Client anger as a predictor of differential response to treatment. In R. Longabaugh & P. W. Wirtz (Eds.), *Project MATCH hypotheses: Results and causal chain analyses* (Vol. 8, pp. 134–148). Bethesda, MD: National Institute on Alcohol Abuse and Alcoholism.

Walthers, J., Janssen, T., Mastroleo, N. R., Hoadley, A., Barnett, N. P., Colby, S. M., & Magill, M. (2019). A sequential analysis of clinician skills and client change statements in a brief motivational intervention for young adult heavy drinking. *Behavior Therapy, 50*(4), 732–742.

Wampold, B. E. (2015). How important are the common factors in psychotherapy?: An update. *World Psychiatry, 14*(3), 270–277.

Wampold, B. E., & Bolt, D. M. (2006). Therapist effects: Clever ways to make them (and everything else) disappear. *Psychotherapy Research, 16*(2), 184–187.

Wampold, B. E., & Brown, G. S. (2005). Estimating variability in outcomes attributable to therapists: A naturalistic study of outcomes in managed care. *Journal of Consulting and Clinical Psychology, 73*(5), 914–923.

Wampold, B. E., & Imel, Z. E. (2015). *The great psychotherapy debate: The evidence for what makes psychotherapy work* (2nd ed.). New York: Routledge.

Wampold, B. E., Minami, T., Tierney, S. C., Baskin, T. W., & Bhati, K. S. (2005). The placebo is powerful: Estimating placebo effects in medicine and psychotherapy from randomized clinical trials. *Journal of Clinical Psychology, 61*(7), 835–854.

Wampold, B. E., & Ulvenes, P. G. (2019). Integration of common factors and specific ingredients. In J. C. Norcross & M. R. Goldfried (Eds.), *Handook of psychotherapy integration* (3rd ed., pp. 69–87). New York: Oxford University Press.

Watson, J. C., & Bedard, D. L. (2006). Clients' emotional processing in psychotherapy: A comparison between cognitive-behavioral and process-experiential therapies. *Journal of Consulting and Clinical Psychology, 74*(1), 152–159.

Watson, J. C., & Greenberg, L. S. (1996). Pathways to change in the psychotherapy of depression: Relating process to session change and outcome. *Psychotherapy, 33,* 262–274.

Watson, J. C., Greenberg, L. S., & Lietaer, G. (1998). The experiential paradigm unfolding: Relationships and experiencing in psychotherapy. In L. S. Greenberg, J. C. Watson, & G. Lietaer (Eds.), *Handbook of experiential psychotherapy* (pp. 3–27). New York: Guilford Press.

Watson, J. C., McMullen, E. J., Rodrigues, A., & Prosser, M. C. (2020). Examining the role of therapists' empathy and clients' attachment styles on changes in clients' affect regulation and outcome in the treatment of depression. *Psychotherapy Research, 30*(6), 693–705.

Webb, C. A., DeRubeis, R. J., & Barber, J. P. (2010). Therapist adherence/competence and treatment outcome: A meta-analytic review. *Journal of Consulting and Clinical Psychology, 78*(2), 200–211.

Weiner, B. (2018). The legacy of an attribution approach to motivation and emotion: A no-crisis zone. *Motivation Science, 4*(1), 4–14.

Weinraub, S. (2018). Presence: The fourth condition. In M. Bazzano (Ed.), *Revisioning person-centred therapy: Theory and practice of a radical paradigm* (pp. 300–314). London: Routledge.

Wells, E. A., Saxon, A. J., Calsyn, D. A., Jackson, T. R., & Donovan, D. M. (2010). Study results from the Clinical Trials Network's first 10 years: Where do they lead? *Journal of Substance Abuse Treatment, 38*(Suppl. 1), S14–S30.

Westerberg, V. S., Miller, W. R., & Tonigan, J. S. (2000). Comparison of outcomes for clients in randomized versus open trials of treatment for alcohol use disorders. *Journal of Studies on Alcohol, 61,* 720–727.

Westermann, R., Spies, K., Stahl, G., & Hesse, F. W. (1996). Relative effectiveness and validity of mood induction procedures: A meta-analysis. *European Journal of Social Psychology, 26*(4), 557–580.

Westra, H. A., Norouzian, N., Poulin, L., Coyne, A., Constantino, M. J., Hara, K., . . . Antony, M. M. (in press). Testing a deliberate practice workshop for developing appropriate responsivity to resistance markers. *Psychotherapy.*

White, W. L., & Miller, W. R. (2007). The use of confrontation in addiction treatment: History, science, and time for a change. *The Counselor, 8*(4), 12–30.

Whitehorn, J. C., & Betz, B. J. (1954, November). A study of psychotherapeutic relationships between physicians and schizophrenic patients. *American Journal of Psychiatry, 111,* 321–331.

Wilkins, P. (2000). Unconditional positive regard reconsidered. *British Journal of Guidance and Counseling, 28*(1), 23–36.

Williams, S. L., & French, D. P. (2011). What are the most effective intervention techniques for changing physical activity self-efficacy and physical activity behaviour–and are they the same? *Health Education Research, 26*(2), 308–322.

Wilson, H. M. N., Davies, J. S., & Weatherhead, S. (2016). Trainee therapists' experiences of supervision during training: A meta-analysis. *Clinical Psychology and Psychotherapy, 23,* 340–351.

Wiser, S. G., & Goldfried, M. R. (1998). Therapist interventions and client emotional experiencing in expert psychodynamic–interpersonal and cognitive-behavioral therapies. *Journal of Consulting and Clinical Psychology, 66*(4), 634–640.

Witkiewitz, K., Bowen, S., Douglas, H., & Hsu, S. H. (2013). Mindfulness-based relapse prevention for substance craving. *Addictive Behaviors, 38*(2), 1563–1571.

Witkiewitz, K., Bowen, S., Harrop, E. N., Douglas, H., Enkema, M., & Sedgwick, C. (2014). Mindfulness-based treatment to prevent addictive behavior relapse: Theoretical models and hypothesized mechanisms of change. *Substance Use and Misuse, 49*(5), 513–524.

Witkiewitz, K., Lustyk, M. K., & Bowen, S. (2013). Retraining the addicted brain: A review of hypothesized neurobiological mechanisms of mindfulness-based relapse prevention. *Psychology of Addictive Behaviors: Journal of the Society of Psychologists in Addictive Behaviors, 27*(2), 351–365.

Witkiewitz, K., & Marlatt, G. A. (2004). Relapse prevention for alcohol and drug problems: That was Zen, this is Tao. *American Psychologist, 59*(4), 224–235.

Witteman, C. L. M., Weiss, D. J., & Metzmacher, M. (2012). Assessing diagnostic expertise of counselors using the Cochran–Weiss–Shanteau (CWS) Index. *Journal of Counseling and Development, 90*(1), 30–34.

Wolf, A. W., Goldfried, M. R., & Muran, J. C. (2017). Therapist negative reactions: How to transform toxic experiences. In L. G. Castonguay & C. Hill (Eds.), *How and why some therapists are better than others: Understanding therapist effects* (pp. 175–192). Washington, DC: American Psychological Association.

Wood, R. E., Mento, A. J., & Locke, E. A. (1987). Task complexity as a moderator of goal effects: A meta-analysis. *Journal of Applied Psychology, 72*(3), 416–425.

Yahne, C. E., & Miller, W. R. (1999). Evoking hope. In W. R. Miller (Ed.), *Integrating spirituality into treatment: Resources for practitioners* (pp. 217–233). Washington, DC: American Psychological Association.

Yalom, I. D. (2002). *The gift of therapy: An open letter to a new generation of therapists and their patients.* New York: HarperCollins.

Zickgraf, H. F., Chambless, D. L., McCarthy, K. S., Gallop, R., Sharpless, B. A., Milrod, B. L., & Barber, J. P. (2016). Interpersonal factors are associated with lower therapist adherence in cognitive-behavioral therapy for panic disorder. *Clinical Psychology and Psychotherapy, 23*(3), 272–284.

Zuroff, D. C., Kelly, A. C., Leybman, M. J., Blatt, S. J., & Wampold, B. E. (2010). Between-therapist and within-therapist differences in the quality of the therapeutic relationship: Effects on maladjustment and self-critical perfectionism. *Journal of Clinical Psychology, 66*(7), 681–697.

Index

Note. f or t following a page number indicates a figure or table.